Nourishing the Gut

A Diverticulitis Cookbook for Flare-Ups and Beyond.

William wright

Copyright

TABLE OF CONTENTS

Introduction

Welcome to "Nourishing the Gut: A Diverticulitis Cookbook for Flare-Ups and Beyond." This cookbook is designed to support you on your journey to managing diverticulitis with ease and confidence. Whether you're navigating a flare-up, recovering, or maintaining digestive health, the recipes and guidance in this book will help you nourish your body while protecting your gut.

As someone who has personally struggled with diverticulitis, I understand the challenges of finding foods that are both gentle on your digestive system and satisfying to your appetite. Over the years, I've learned how food choices can play a crucial role in managing symptoms and preventing flare-ups. This cookbook is a culmination of my own healing journey, along with extensive research, trial and error, and consultations with nutrition experts. It is my hope that these recipes provide relief, support, and encouragement for those navigating this condition.

The purpose of this book is to offer practical, delicious, and healing recipes tailored to each phase of diverticulitis. From liquid diets during flare-ups to high-fiber meals for long-term maintenance, you'll find everything you need to cook meals that are both gut-friendly and nourishing. Together, we'll explore the power of food in managing diverticulitis and empowering you to live well.

Understanding Diverticulitis and Diverticulosis

Diverticulosis and diverticulitis are two conditions that affect the digestive tract, specifically the colon. While they are related, they differ significantly in terms of symptoms, severity, and the management required. Understanding these conditions, along with how diet plays a vital role in managing flare-ups and promoting healing, can help individuals with diverticular disease live more comfortably and effectively manage their symptoms.

Diverticulosis is the presence of small, bulging pouches (called diverticula) that form in the walls of the colon. These pouches develop when weak spots in the colon wall give way under pressure, causing small pockets to form. Diverticulosis often occurs with age and is common in individuals over 40. In most cases, diverticulosis does not cause symptoms and may only be discovered during routine colonoscopies or imaging tests. This condition is often asymptomatic, but it can be managed with lifestyle changes, particularly a diet rich in fiber. Fiber helps soften stools and prevent constipation, which reduces the risk of diverticula forming or becoming inflamed.

Diverticulitis, on the other hand, occurs when one or more of these diverticula become inflamed or infected. This can happen when food particles, stool, or bacteria get trapped inside a diverticulum, causing irritation and infection. Diverticulitis is often more serious than diverticulosis and requires medical treatment. A flare-up can result in severe pain, fever, nausea, and changes in bowel movements. In severe cases, diverticulitis can lead to complications such as abscesses, perforations (holes in the colon), bleeding, or peritonitis (infection of the abdominal cavity). Treatment often involves antibiotics, and in some cases, surgery may be necessary to remove the affected portion of the colon.

Symptoms of Diverticulitis

The symptoms of diverticulitis can range from mild to severe, depending on the extent of inflammation or infection. Common symptoms include:

Abdominal pain: The most common symptom of diverticulitis is sharp, crampy pain, typically in the lower left side of the abdomen. However, the pain may also occur in other areas depending on which part of the colon is affected.

Fever: A fever is a common sign of infection and may be accompanied by chills.

Nausea and vomiting: These symptoms often occur due to the body's response to pain and infection.

Changes in bowel movements: Diarrhea or constipation may develop, and some individuals may notice blood in their stools.

Bloating and cramping: A feeling of fullness, bloating, or tenderness in the abdomen is also common during a flare-up.

It's important to seek medical attention if you experience any of these symptoms, especially if they persist or worsen over time. A healthcare provider can diagnose the condition through imaging tests and determine the appropriate treatment plan.

Causes of Diverticulitis

While the exact cause of diverticulitis is not entirely understood, several factors contribute to the development of diverticulosis and the subsequent risk of diverticulitis. These include:

Age: As people age, the colon weakens and becomes more prone to the formation of diverticula. The risk increases after age 40, with the likelihood rising significantly in those over 60.

Diet: A low-fiber diet is a major contributing factor to the development of diverticulosis. When the diet lacks fiber, stools become harder and more difficult to pass, leading to increased pressure in the colon. Over time, this pressure can cause the weak spots in the colon to form pouches (diverticula).

Constipation: Straining during bowel movements, often due to constipation, can put additional pressure on the colon walls, making diverticula more likely to form.

Obesity: Being overweight increases the risk of diverticulitis. The excess fat may place additional pressure on the digestive system, increasing the likelihood of inflammation and infection in the diverticula.

Common Triggers of Diverticulitis

Several factors may trigger or exacerbate diverticulitis, particularly during a flare-up. Understanding these triggers is essential for managing the condition effectively:

Low-fiber diet: One of the most significant contributors to diverticulitis flare-ups is a low-fiber diet. Without enough fiber to bulk up stool and promote regular bowel movements, the colon can become congested, leading to increased pressure and irritation in the diverticula. This can contribute to inflammation and infection in the colon. A diet high in fiber, particularly soluble fiber, is essential for preventing flare-ups and promoting long-term digestive health.

Certain foods: While some older recommendations advised avoiding foods like nuts, seeds, and popcorn due to concerns that they might get stuck in diverticula, recent research suggests that these foods are generally safe for individuals with diverticulosis and diverticulitis. However, high-fat, spicy, or processed foods can irritate the digestive tract and trigger symptoms, so it's wise to limit their consumption during flare-ups.

Constipation: Chronic constipation can lead to straining during bowel movements, which increases pressure on the colon and may contribute to the development of diverticula. It's essential to maintain regular bowel movements by consuming enough fiber and drinking plenty of water.

Obesity: Being overweight or obese increases the risk of diverticulitis and may worsen flare-ups. Maintaining a healthy weight through diet and exercise can help reduce the likelihood of diverticulitis episodes.

Medications: Certain medications, such as nonsteroidal anti-inflammatory drugs (NSAIDs), opioids, and corticosteroids, may increase the risk of diverticulitis flare-ups by affecting the gut and bowel function.

Importance of Diet in Managing Flare-Ups and Promoting Healing

Diet plays a crucial role in both preventing and managing diverticulitis. During a flare-up, a low-residue or liquid diet is often recommended to allow the colon to heal and reduce strain on the digestive system. Foods that are easy to digest and low in fiber, such as clear broths, white rice, and applesauce, can help minimize irritation. Once symptoms begin to subside, soft, low-fiber foods are gradually reintroduced to help the body recover without overstressing the gut.

After the flare-up has resolved, a high-fiber diet becomes critical for preventing future episodes. Fiber helps to soften stools, reduce constipation, and maintain regular bowel movements, all of which help to prevent pressure buildup in the colon. A diet rich in fiber from fruits, vegetables, whole grains, and legumes is essential for long-term digestive health.

In addition to fiber, anti-inflammatory foods such as omega-3 rich fish, turmeric, and ginger can help promote healing and reduce inflammation in the digestive tract. Staying hydrated is also essential, as water helps keep stools soft and prevents constipation.

A well-balanced diet, rich in fiber and anti-inflammatory foods, is a cornerstone of managing diverticulitis, supporting healing during flare-ups, and preventing future complications. By focusing on a gut-friendly diet, individuals with diverticulitis can significantly improve their quality of life and reduce the frequency and severity of flare-ups.

Nutrition Essentials for Diverticulitis

Proper nutrition plays a critical role in managing diverticulitis and promoting healing. Understanding which foods are beneficial and which may trigger flare-ups can help individuals with diverticulitis maintain digestive health, prevent complications, and reduce the frequency of attacks.

1. High-Quality Protein

Protein is essential for tissue repair and immune function, especially during and after a diverticulitis flare-up. Lean sources of protein, such as skinless poultry, fish, eggs, tofu, and legumes, provide the building blocks necessary for healing and maintaining muscle mass. When the digestive system is in distress, opt for well-cooked or pureed forms of protein for easier digestion.

Tip: Include soft-cooked eggs or blended tofu in your meals to support digestion during flare-ups.

2. Fiber: Balancing Soluble and Insoluble

Fiber is a key element in maintaining digestive health, but it needs to be consumed thoughtfully in the case of diverticulitis. During a flare-up, a low-fiber or liquid diet is often recommended to reduce irritation in the intestines. Once symptoms subside, gradually increasing fiber intake from plant-based foods can help prevent constipation and ease digestion.

- Soluble fiber (found in oats, apples, and carrots) absorbs water, forming a gel-like substance that helps regulate bowel movements and reduce inflammation.

- Insoluble fiber (found in whole grains, nuts, and raw vegetables) adds bulk to stool but can irritate the digestive system during a flare-up. Once you're in remission, slowly reintroduce these foods to support regularity.

Tip: Start with cooked or canned vegetables and soft fruits for easy digestion, then gradually reintroduce higher-fiber foods like whole grains.

3. Hydration

Proper hydration is vital for digestive health, particularly when managing diverticulitis. Drinking enough water ensures that stool remains soft and easy to pass, reducing the risk of constipation, which can contribute to diverticulitis flare-ups. Staying hydrated also aids in nutrient absorption and helps your body recover from the inflammation that often accompanies a flare.

Tip: Aim for at least 8 glasses of water daily, and consider drinking herbal teas or broths to keep your hydration levels up.

4. Healthy Fats

Healthy fats, such as those from avocados, olive oil, and nuts (in moderation), are important for maintaining cellular function and overall well-being. Omega-3 fatty acids found in fatty fish (salmon, mackerel) and flaxseeds also have anti-inflammatory properties that may help reduce the inflammation associated with diverticulitis.

Tip: Include a small serving of fatty fish a few times a week to boost omega-3 intake for its anti-inflammatory benefits.

5. Limit Processed and Red Meat

Processed foods and red meats are typically high in unhealthy fats and can worsen inflammation in the body. To promote gut health, limit your intake of red meat, processed meats (such as bacon, sausage, and deli meats), and refined sugars. These foods can trigger flare-ups or exacerbate existing symptoms.

Tip: Choose lean cuts of meat and plant-based protein sources to reduce inflammation and support digestive function.

By focusing on a balanced dict that prioritizes lean proteins, fiber, hydration, healthy fats, and limited processed foods, individuals with diverticulitis can manage their symptoms more effectively and promote long-term digestive health.

Lifestyle Tips for Digestive Health

Managing diverticulitis and maintaining digestive health requires more than just a balanced diet. Lifestyle changes that support gut health can prevent flare-ups, reduce inflammation, and promote overall well-being. Adopting the following tips can help individuals with diverticulitis lead a healthier, more comfortable life.

1. Stay Active

Regular physical activity is essential for digestive health. Exercise helps stimulate the intestines, promoting regular bowel movements and preventing constipation, a key risk factor for diverticulitis flare-ups. Aim for at least 30 minutes of moderate exercise most days of the week. Activities like walking, swimming, or cycling are gentle on the body and can significantly improve gastrointestinal function.

Tips:

- Start slowly if you're not already active, and gradually increase the intensity and duration of your exercise.

- Avoid intense workouts during a diverticulitis flare-up to prevent added stress on the body.

2. Maintain a Healthy Weight

Obesity is a risk factor for diverticulitis, as excess weight can increase pressure on the digestive system. Maintaining a healthy weight through balanced eating and regular exercise helps reduce the likelihood of flare-ups and supports overall digestive health. Aiming for gradual, sustainable weight loss through lifestyle changes is often more effective than fad diets.

Tips:

- Focus on portion control and eating nutrient-dense foods, such as vegetables, fruits, whole grains, and lean proteins.

- Avoid crash dieting, which can stress the body and negatively impact gut function.

3. Stay Hydrated

Drinking plenty of water is essential for good digestive health. Staying well-hydrated helps keep stools soft, preventing constipation and the associated pressure on the colon. It also helps support the digestion of fiber, making it easier for the body to process and absorb nutrients.

Tips:

- Aim for at least 8 glasses of water per day, more if you're physically active or live in a hot climate.

- Herbal teas and broths can also be hydrating and soothing for the digestive system.

4. Manage Stress

Stress can exacerbate digestive problems, including diverticulitis. High levels of stress can disrupt the digestive system, increase inflammation, and lead to poor dietary choices. Incorporating stress management techniques into your daily routine can promote better gut health and overall well-being.

Tips:

- Practice relaxation techniques such as deep breathing, yoga, or meditation to help reduce stress levels.

- Consider journaling or talking with a counselor to address any emotional challenges that may affect your digestion.

5. Avoid Smoking and Limit Alcohol

Smoking and excessive alcohol consumption can irritate the digestive tract and worsen symptoms of diverticulitis. Smoking, in particular, can increase the risk of inflammation, slow down digestion, and make it harder for the body to heal during a flare-up. Alcohol can cause dehydration and irritate the gut lining.

Tips:

- If you smoke, consider seeking support to quit, such as nicotine replacement therapy or counseling.

- Limit alcohol intake to one drink per day or avoid it altogether, e.specially during flare-ups.

6. Avoid Straining During Bowel Movements

Straining during bowel movements puts extra pressure on the colon, which can worsen diverticulitis symptoms and lead to more diverticula forming. Ensuring smooth, regular bowel movements is essential for preventing flare-ups. A diet high in fiber and sufficient hydration can prevent constipation, which is a major cause of straining.

Tips:

- Don't rush when using the bathroom—take your time to allow for a natural bowel movement.

- Use a footstool or squatty potty to elevate your feet while sitting on the toilet. This position can make it easier to pass stools without straining.

7. Get Enough Sleep

Good sleep is essential for overall health, including digestive health. Poor sleep can disrupt gut function and contribute to inflammation, making it harder for the body to heal. Aim for 7–9 hours of quality sleep each night to allow your body to rest and recover.

Tips:

- Establish a regular bedtime routine to improve sleep quality, such as avoiding screens before bed, creating a calm sleep environment, and sticking to a consistent sleep schedule.

- If you have trouble sleeping, try relaxing activities like reading or a warm bath before bed.

8. Monitor Your Fiber Intake

Fiber is crucial for maintaining digestive health, but the type and amount of fiber you consume should be adjusted depending on whether you're experiencing a diverticulitis flare-up or not. During a flare-up, a low-fiber or liquid diet may be recommended, but once you're in remission, a high-fiber diet helps prevent constipation and reduces pressure on the colon.

Tips:

- During flare-ups, focus on easily digestible, low-residue foods like broth, white rice, and cooked vegetables.

- Once symptoms subside, gradually reintroduce high-fiber foods such as whole grains, fruits, vegetables, and legumes to support regular bowel movements.

9. Avoid Overeating

Eating large meals can put unnecessary strain on the digestive system and increase the risk of symptoms such as bloating and discomfort. Opt for smaller, more frequent meals throughout the day to reduce the workload on your digestive tract.

Tips:

- Divide your daily food intake into smaller meals—around 4–6 meals a day rather than three large ones.

- Avoid overeating, especially at night, to allow for easier digestion before bed.

10. Follow Your Doctor's Advice

Lastly, it's essential to work with your healthcare provider to manage diverticulitis effectively. Follow your doctor's guidance regarding medications, dietary restrictions, and lifestyle changes. Regular check-ups are also crucial to monitor the condition and prevent complications.

Tlps:

- Keep a food diary to track what you eat and any symptoms you experience, helping you and your healthcare provider make informed decisions about your diet and treatment.

- Don't hesitate to ask your doctor for recommendations on managing symptoms or preventing flare-ups.

By adopting these lifestyle habits, you can support your digestive health, reduce the risk of diverticulitis flare-ups, and promote healing. A combination of a balanced diet, regular exercise, hydration, stress management, and preventive measures will help you manage diverticulitis and improve your quality of life.

Chapter 1

Nourishing the Gut

In managing diverticulitis, one of the most important steps is ensuring that your diet supports your digestive system. Whether you're in the midst of a flare-up or looking to prevent future ones, your food choices play a significant role in how your gut functions and heals. The right foods can help reduce inflammation, promote healing, and keep your digestive system running smoothly. On the other hand, the wrong foods—especially during a flare-up—can exacerbate symptoms and delay recovery.

This chapter provides helpful shopping lists to guide you in selecting foods that support your gut health at different stages of diverticulitis. Whether you're following a low-fiber diet during an acute flare-up or gradually reintroducing fiber-rich foods after recovery, these lists offer a structured approach to eating that promotes healing and long-term digestive health. By making mindful food choices, you'll not only nourish your gut but also set yourself up for better overall health and well-being.

Shopping Lists for Digestive Health

A balanced, nutrient-dense diet is essential for managing diverticulitis and supporting gut health. When you're dealing with diverticulitis, it can be challenging to know what foods to buy and what to avoid. This chapter offers detailed shopping lists to help you make healthier food choices, support digestion, and minimize the risk of flare-ups. Whether you are experiencing a flare-up or in remission, this guide provides the foundation for nourishing your digestive system.

Shopping for a Low-Fiber Diet (During a Flare-Up)

During a diverticulitis flare-up, a low-fiber or liquid diet may be recommended to reduce irritation in the digestive tract. The goal is to give your intestines time to heal while still providing the necessary nutrients. Foods should be soft, easy to digest, and non-irritating.

Fruits and Vegetables (Cooked and Peeled)

When in a flare-up, you'll want to avoid high-fiber fruits and vegetables, especially raw ones. Stick to cooked and peeled fruits and vegetables, which are easier to digest and gentler on your intestines. Aim for small portions of these foods:

- Cooked carrots

- Cooked potatoes (peeled)

- Applesauce (unsweetened)

- Canned peaches or pears (in their own juice, no syrup)

- Bananas (ripe and soft)

- Cucumber (peeled)

- Zucchini (peeled)

Protein Sources

During flare-ups, protein intake is important for tissue repair and overall health, but it should come from lean and easily digestible sources. Avoid red meats and high-fat proteins, opting instead for softer, lower-fat options:

- Lean poultry (chicken or turkey)

- Fish (white fish like cod, tilapia, or salmon)

- Eggs (scrambled or soft-boiled)

- Tofu (silken)

- Low-fat cottage cheese

- Plain Greek yogurt (unsweetened)

Grains and Carbohydrates

Avoid whole grains and high-fiber foods during a flare-up, as they can irritate the colon. Stick to refined grains and low-fiber carbohydrates that are gentle on your digestive system:

- White rice

- Refined pasta

- Plain white bread

- Cream of wheat

- Oatmeal (smooth or well-cooked)

Dairy and Alternatives

Dairy can sometimes be an issue during flare-ups, especially if you are lactose intolerant. Choose low-fat or lactose-free alternatives to avoid unnecessary irritation:

- Lactose-free milk

- Low-fat or lactose-free yogurt

- Almond milk (unsweetened)

- Coconut milk (unsweetened)

Soups and Broths

Clear liquids are often recommended during a flare-up for hydration and digestive rest. Broths and soups without high-fiber vegetables are great options:

- Chicken or vegetable broth

- Clear consommé

- Broth-based soups (strained)

- Plain cream soups (without added vegetables or meat)

Other Essentials

Other items to stock up on for a low-fiber diet during a flare-up include easy-to-digest, non-irritating foods:

- White crackers

- Plain noodles (refined, not whole grain)

- Gelatin (unsweetened)

- Smooth peanut butter (without added sugar or salt)

- Honey or maple syrup (in moderation)

Shopping for a High-Fiber Diet (Post-Flare-Up or Maintenance)

Once your symptoms subside, it's important to gradually reintroduce fiber-rich foods to help maintain healthy digestion and prevent future flare-ups. A high-fiber diet promotes regular bowel movements, reduces constipation, and supports overall colon health. However, it's important to increase fiber slowly to avoid overwhelming your digestive system.

Fruits and Vegetables

Incorporate a variety of high-fiber fruits and vegetables into your diet. These foods are packed with vitamins, minerals, and antioxidants, as well as soluble and insoluble fiber:

- Apples (with skin)

- Pears (with skin)

- Berries (strawberries, blueberries, raspberries)

- Carrots (raw or lightly cooked)

- Broccoli (steamed or raw)

- Spinach (raw or lightly sautéed)

- Sweet potatoes (with skin)

- Squash (butternut, acorn)

- Leafy greens (kale, arugula, swiss chard)

Whole Grains

Whole grains provide both soluble and insoluble fiber, which help keep your digestive system running smoothly. These foods also provide essential vitamins, minerals, and antioxidants:

- Whole wheat bread

- Brown rice

- Whole wheat pasta

- Oats (steel-cut or rolled oats)

- Quinoa

- Barley

- Farro

- Whole grain cereals (unsweetened)

Legumes

Legumes are rich in fiber, protein, and healthy carbohydrates. These should be reintroduced gradually and in small portions if your digestive system is sensitive. Well-cooked beans and lentils can help support digestion:

- Lentils (well-cooked)

- Black beans

- Chickpeas

- Kidney beans

- Peas

- Edamame (young soybeans)

Healthy Fats

Incorporating healthy fats into your diet can help reduce inflammation and promote nutrient absorption. Choose sources of unsaturated fats, which are beneficial for gut health:

- Avocados

- Olive oil

- Nuts (almonds, walnuts, cashews)

- Nut butters (smooth, unsweetened)

- Chia seeds and flaxseeds

Dairy and Alternatives

If you tolerate dairy, include it as a source of calcium and protein. Opt for low-fat versions or plant-based alternatives:

- Low-fat milk

- Greek yogurt (unsweetened)

- Almond or soy milk (unsweetened)

- Cheese (in moderation)

Herbs and Spices

Herbs and spices not only enhance the flavor of your meals but can also support digestion and reduce inflammation. Use them to season your food instead of relying on salt:

- Ginger

- Turmeric

- Cilantro

- Basil

- Oregano

- Thyme

Additional Tips for Shopping and Meal Prep

Plan your meals. Having a weekly meal plan can help ensure you get the right balance of nutrients. It will also help you avoid impulse purchases of foods that might irritate your gut.

Read food labels: Always check for added sugars, excessive sodium, or artificial ingredients in packaged foods. Opt for whole, minimally processed options.

Batch cook: Prepare and freeze meals in advance so you always have a healthy option on hand, especially during flare-ups.

With these shopping lists and tips, you can create a digestive-friendly meal plan tailored to your needs. Whether you're managing a flare-up or looking to maintain gut health long-term, nourishing your body with the right foods is essential for healing and overall well-being.

Techniques for preparing easy-to-digest foods

When managing diverticulitis, preparing your meals in a way that makes them easier on the digestive system is key. The method of preparation can significantly impact how well your body tolerates certain foods. This section provides various techniques to make foods easier to digest, whether you are in the middle of a flare-up or working to prevent one. These cooking methods can help minimize irritation in the digestive tract while maximizing nutrient absorption.

1. Peeling and Removing Skins

Many fruits and vegetables contain a high amount of fiber in their skins, which can be hard to digest, especially during a flare-up. Peeling your produce can help reduce its fiber content and make it gentler on the stomach. Here are some common foods to peel:

- Apples and pears: While they are rich in fiber, their skins can be tough to digest. Peel them before eating to reduce fiber content.

- Cucumbers: The skin of cucumbers can be harsh on the stomach. Peel them before adding them to salads or dishes.

- Potatoes: While potato skins are a good source of fiber, removing them makes them easier to digest, especially when boiled or mashed.

- Tomatoes: Remove the skin of tomatoes before adding them to sauces or salads to make them gentler on your digestive system.

2. Pureeing

Pureeing is a great technique for making foods easier to digest, as it breaks down the food into smaller particles that are more easily absorbed by the body. This method is especially helpful for fruits, vegetables, and grains that can be tough on the digestive system when eaten whole or in chunks.

- Vegetables: Steamed or boiled vegetables can be pureed into soups or sauces. Carrots, sweet potatoes, and squash all puree well and are packed with nutrients.

- Fruits: Fruits like bananas, berries, and apples can be pureed into smoothies or applesauce. This makes them easier to digest and provides a refreshing, soothing option during flare-ups.

- Soups: Consider pureeing your soups to remove any potential chunks of fiber. Blending ingredients such as carrots, peas, and tomatoes helps create a smooth, easy-to-digest base.

3. Steaming

Steaming is a gentle cooking method that helps retain nutrients while making foods softer and easier to digest. Unlike boiling, which can leach out nutrients, steaming keeps the food's vitamins and minerals intact.

- Vegetables: Steaming vegetables like carrots, zucchini, and broccoli softens them, making them much easier to tolerate. It also helps preserve their nutrients, so you get the maximum benefit from each serving.

- Fish: Steaming fish makes it tender and moist without the need for oils or fats that might be hard on the stomach.

- Chicken and Poultry: Steaming chicken breasts or turkey makes them softer and less dry, which can make them easier to digest compared to frying or grilling.

4. Boiling or Poaching

Both boiling and poaching involve cooking food in water or broth, which helps soften it and break down fibers, making it easier on the digestive system. These techniques work especially well for foods like poultry, eggs, and root vegetables.

- Eggs: Soft-boiling or poaching eggs keeps them tender and easy to digest. They are a gentle protein source for those experiencing digestive distress.

- Chicken and Fish: Boiling chicken or fish in a light broth helps break down the proteins, making them easier to digest while still retaining moisture and flavor.

- Vegetables: Boiling root vegetables like carrots, sweet potatoes, and beets can soften their fibers and make them gentler on the stomach. Avoid overcooking, as this can make some vegetables mushy and less appealing.

5. Grinding or Mashing

For those with sensitive digestive systems, grinding or mashing food into smaller pieces can be a game-changer. This process reduces the effort required by the digestive system and makes it easier for the body to break down and absorb nutrients.

- Meat: Ground meats, such as chicken, turkey, or lean beef, are easier to digest than whole cuts of meat. You can use ground meat in soups, stews, or casseroles, where it can be easily mixed with other ingredients.

- Potatoes: Mashed potatoes (without the skin) are soft and easy to digest. You can make them smoother by adding small amounts of broth or low-fat milk to achieve the desired consistency.

- Rice: When cooking rice, make sure it's fully cooked and soft. If needed, you can mash it or blend it into a smoother texture, making it gentler on the digestive system.

6. Cooking in Broth

Cooking in broth instead of water can add extra flavor and nutrients to your food while keeping it moist and easy to swallow. The liquid helps to soften foods and make them easier to digest, especially for people who are experiencing difficulty swallowing or chewing.

- Vegetables: Cooking vegetables like zucchini, carrots, and peas in broth helps them stay moist and tender. It can also add extra flavor without the need for heavy seasoning or spices.

- **Meats:** Simmering meat in broth ensures it stays tender and soft. This is a great option for lean cuts of beef, chicken, or turkey.

- **Grains:** Cooking rice, quinoa, or barley in broth can make them more flavorful and easier to eat when you have a sensitive stomach.

7. Avoiding High-Heat Methods (Grilling, Frying, Roasting)

While grilling, frying, and roasting are popular cooking methods, they can cause food to become tough, dry, or overly caramelized, which can be difficult for your digestive system to handle. These high-heat techniques should generally be avoided during a flare-up or when trying to follow a gentle, easy-to-digest diet.

Instead, opt for gentle cooking methods like steaming, boiling, poaching, or slow-cooking. These methods ensure your food remains soft, moist, and easy to digest, minimizing the risk of irritation to the gut.

Incorporating these techniques into your meal preparation will help ensure that the foods you eat are easy to digest and gentle on your gut. By choosing the right cooking methods, you can support your digeslive system, reduce discomfort, and promote healing while enjoying nutritious and satisfying meals.

Chapter 2

Flare-Up Phase Recipes

During a diverticulitis flare-up, your body is inflamed and needs extra care and rest, especially in terms of diet. Eating the right foods during this phase can significantly impact your recovery, as it helps reduce inflammation, ease digestive discomfort, and allow the digestive tract to heal. In this chapter, you'll find recipes specifically tailored to be gentle on your system, low in fiber, and easy to digest.

These recipes focus on nourishing, simple ingredients that won't stress your digestive system while still providing essential nutrients. From soothing broths to pureed soups and hydrating smoothies, these options are crafted to give your body the support it needs without aggravating symptoms.

The goal of this chapter is to offer a selection of recipes that are safe and beneficial during a flare-up, keeping your digestive system at ease and encouraging a quicker, more comfortable recovery.

42

By following these meal suggestions, you can nourish yourself gently, rebuild strength, and gradually move toward foods that support your healing journey.

The flare-up phase of diverticulitis is a period of acute inflammation, pain, and sensitivity in the digestive system. During this time, the lining of the intestines is inflamed, which can lead to significant discomfort, cramping, and digestive distress. This phase often requires careful dietary adjustments to reduce irritation and allow the body to heal. Understanding how to manage this stage is essential for minimizing symptoms and speeding up recovery.

Diet plays a critical role during a flare-up. While the inflammation is active, the digestive system needs foods that are easy to digest and low in fiber. A low-fiber diet can help prevent further irritation to the intestinal walls and allow the digestive tract to rest and recover. This approach includes consuming clear liquids, such as broths and hydrating drinks, and gradually introducing gentle, low-fiber foods like pureed soups, cooked vegetables, and lean proteins as the symptoms begin to improve.

In addition to dietary changes, hydration is essential during a flare-up. Drinking plenty of fluids helps prevent dehydration, particularly if symptoms like nausea or reduced appetite occur. As your body heals, listening to its signals and introducing foods slowly can ease the transition and prevent additional discomfort. The flare-up phase is challenging, but with the right foods and care, you can support your recovery and move closer to regaining digestive health.

Low-residue Diets and Liquid options for Flare-ups

During a diverticulitis flare-up, a low-residue diet is recommended to reduce strain on the digestive tract. "Residue" refers to the indigestible parts of food, especially fiber, that can accumulate in the intestines. A low-residue diet minimizes these residues, which helps to reduce irritation, cramping, and discomfort during a flare-up. This approach focuses on foods that are easy to digest and pass through the digestive system smoothly, reducing the workload on inflamed areas.

In the early stages of a flare-up, a clear liquid diet is often recommended to give the digestive system complete rest. Clear liquids include options such as broth, gelatin, herbal teas, apple juice, and electrolyte drinks. These provide hydration and some nutrients without introducing fiber or solids, allowing inflamed tissues to begin healing without added stress.

As symptoms gradually improve, low-residue solid foods can be slowly introduced. This phase might include foods like white rice, plain pasta, mashed potatoes without skins, and skinless, well-cooked vegetables (such as carrots or zucchini). Protein sources like eggs, soft-cooked chicken, and fish are also ideal for this stage, as they provide essential nutrients while being gentle on the digestive system. Avoid high-fiber foods like raw vegetables, seeds, nuts, and whole grains until symptoms fully subside.

Both low-residue diets and liquid options provide crucial support during a flare-up by reducing digestive stress and promoting a smoother recovery. By following these dietary guidelines and progressing gradually, you can help minimize symptoms, reduce inflammation, and encourage healing during this delicate phase.

Hydrating Beverages

Staying hydrated is essential during a diverticulitis flare-up, as dehydration can worsen symptoms and delay recovery. Hydration helps soothe the digestive tract, reduce inflammation, and prevent constipation, which is crucial when following a low-residue diet. Here are some gentle, hydrating beverage options to support you during a flare-up:

1. Water

Plain water is the best source of hydration and should be your primary choice. Aim to drink small, frequent sips throughout the day rather than large amounts at once, especially if nausea is present.

2. Electrolyte Drinks

Electrolyte drinks, like those with low sugar and added electrolytes (such as potassium, sodium, and magnesium), can help replenish lost minerals and prevent dehydration, especially if you're experiencing nausea or diarrhea. Look for options without added sugars or artificial colors.

3. Herbal Teas

Herbal teas, particularly ginger, chamomile, and peppermint, can be soothing to the digestive tract. Ginger tea can help reduce nausea, while chamomile and peppermint have calming effects. Avoid teas with caffeine, as they may irritate the digestive system.

4. Broth

Clear broths, such as vegetable, chicken, or bone broth, provide hydration and essential nutrients like sodium and potassium. Broth is also a comforting, nourishing option for maintaining hydration while giving your digestive system a break from solids.

5. Diluted Fruit Juices

Diluted apple, grape, or cranberry juice can provide hydration with a bit of natural sugar for energy. Make sure to dilute these juices with water to reduce their acidity and sugar concentration, which makes them easier on the stomach.

These hydrating beverages offer gentle, effective ways to support your body through a flare-up, helping to reduce inflammation and promote healing.

Bone Broth with Ginger

Bone broth with ginger is a soothing and nutritious option for those experiencing a diverticulitis flare-up. Bone broth provides essential nutrients like collagen, amino acids, and minerals that support healing, while ginger offers anti-inflammatory and digestive-soothing benefits.

Ingredients

- 4 cups of bone broth (chicken or beef)

- 1-inch piece of fresh ginger, peeled and sliced

- 1 garlic clove, peeled (optional)

- 1-2 teaspoons apple cider vinegar (optional, helps draw nutrients from the bones)

- Salt to taste (if needed)

Instructions

1. In a saucepan, combine the bone broth, sliced ginger, and garlic (if using).

2. Bring to a simmer over medium heat and allow it to simmer gently for 10-15 minutes to infuse the flavors.

3. Remove from heat and strain out the ginger and garlic if you prefer a smoother broth.

4. Add a teaspoon of apple cider vinegar for additional nutrients (optional).

5. Season with a pinch of salt if desired.

Serving Suggestions

Sip on this warm broth slowly. The ginger in the broth may help reduce nausea and calm digestive discomfort. This simple yet nourishing beverage can be enjoyed any time during a flare-up to provide gentle, hydrating nutrition and aid in digestion.

Electrolyte Infused Water

Electrolyte-infused water can help replenish lost minerals and keep you hydrated during a flare-up. These gentle, refreshing recipes use natural ingredients that add subtle flavor and essential electrolytes without any added sugars or artificial ingredients.

Cucumber Mint Electrolyte Water

Ingredients:

- 1/2 cucumber, thinly sliced

- 6-8 fresh mint leaves

- 1/4 teaspoon Himalayan or sea salt (for electrolytes)

- 1 quart (4 cups) filtered water

Instructions:

1. In a large pitcher, combine the cucumber slices, mint leaves, and salt.

2. Pour in the water and stir well.

3. Let it sit in the fridge for at least 1 hour to allow the flavors to infuse.

4. Serve chilled, stirring gently before pouring.

Lemon Ginger Electrolyte Water

Ingredients:

- 1/2 lemon, thinly sliced

- 1-inch piece of fresh ginger, sliced

- 1/4 teaspoon Himalayan or sea salt (for electrolytes)

- 1 quart (4 cups) filtered water

Instructions:

1. In a large pitcher, combine the lemon slices, ginger, and salt.

2. Add the water and stir.

3. Refrigerate for at least 1 hour to infuse flavors.

4. Serve chilled, stirring before pouring.

Both of these infused water recipes offer refreshing flavors with natural electrolytes from the added salt. Sip on them throughout the day to stay hydrated and maintain essential mineral levels.

Chamomile and Peppermint Herbal Teas

Chamomile and peppermint teas are gentle, caffeine-free options that can be especially soothing during a diverticulitis flare-up. Both teas help calm the digestive tract and reduce inflammation, offering relief from discomfort and aiding in relaxation.

Chamomile Tea

Chamomile tea is known for its calming effects on both the mind and the digestive system. It may help reduce cramping and bloating, making it ideal for sensitive stomachs.

Ingredients:

- 1 chamomile tea bag (or 1 tablespoon dried chamomile flowers)

- 1 cup boiling water

- Honey (optional)

Instructions:

1. Place the chamomile tea bag or dried flowers in a cup.

2. Pour boiling water over the tea and let it steep for 5–7 minutes.

3. Remove the tea bag or strain the flowers. Add honey if desired.

4. Sip slowly and enjoy the soothing effects.

Peppermint Tea

Peppermint tea is refreshing and has natural anti-spasmodic properties, which can help relax the digestive muscles and alleviate bloating or nausea.

Ingredients:

- 1 peppermint tea bag (or 1 tablespoon dried peppermint leaves)

- 1 cup boiling water

- Honey (optional)

Instructions:

1. Place the peppermint tea bag or dried leaves in a cup.

2. Pour boiling water over the tea and let it steep for 5–7 minutes.

3. Remove the tea bag or strain the leaves. Add honey if desired.

4. Sip slowly, allowing the tea to soothe any digestive discomfort.

These herbal teas can be enjoyed anytime during the day to promote hydration and provide gentle relief from digestive issues.

Soups and Broths

Soups and broths are excellent choices for managing digestive sensitivity, especially during a diverticulitis flare-up. They are easy to digest, provide essential nutrients, and help maintain hydration. Here are a few nourishing soup and broth recipes tailored for digestive health, featuring gentle ingredients and soothing flavors.

Benefits of Soups and Broths

1. Easy to Digest: Soups and broths are typically soft, making them easy on the digestive system.

2. Hydration: Liquid-based meals help keep the body hydrated, especially when digestive health issues may lead to dehydration.

3. Nutrient-Dense: Soups and broths can be packed with essential vitamins and minerals, particularly when prepared with nutrient-rich ingredients like vegetables and bone broth.

4. Anti-Inflammatory Ingredients: Ingredients like ginger, carrots, and turmeric have anti-inflammatory properties that may help reduce inflammation in the digestive tract.

Recipes

1. Clear Vegetable Broth

A light and nutrient-rich broth made with carrots, celery, and a touch of ginger, this vegetable broth is soothing and hydrating.

Ingredients: Carrots, celery, ginger, parsley, salt, and water.

Instructions: Simmer ingredients until vegetables are soft. Strain and sip the clear broth.

2. Carrot and Ginger Soup (Strained)

Carrots and ginger provide a gentle flavor, while the strained consistency makes it suitable for sensitive stomachs.

Ingredients: Carrots, ginger, potato (optional), vegetable broth, and salt.

Instructions: Sauté carrots and ginger, add broth, simmer until soft, and blend until smooth. Strain if necessary.

3. Bone Broth with Ginger

Bone broth is rich in collagen and amino acids that support gut health. Adding ginger can soothe inflammation and calm nausea.

Ingredients: Bone broth, fresh ginger, garlic, and salt.

Instructions: Simmer ginger and garlic in the broth for added flavor. Strain and enjoy warm.

4. Potato and Leek Puree (Liquid Consistency)

Potatoes and leeks make a creamy, mild soup that's gentle on digestion when blended to a liquid consistency.

Ingredients: Potatoes, leeks, vegetable broth, olive oil, and salt.

Instructions: Sauté leeks, add potatoes and broth, simmer, blend, and thin to a liquid consistency.

Tips for Enjoying Soups and Broths

- Serve Warm: Warm temperatures are often more soothing than hot or cold.

- Strain if Needed: For sensitive stomachs, strain the soup to remove any remaining solids.

- Add Natural Electrolytes: A pinch of sea salt can add electrolytes, especially helpful during a flare-up.

Soups and broths are versatile and comforting meal options, allowing for easy adjustments to flavor and consistency, while promoting gentle, nutrient-rich nourishment during digestive sensitivity phases.

Strained Vegetable Broth with Parsley

This Strained Vegetable Broth with Parsley is a gentle, clear broth designed to be soothing and easy to digest, perfect for flare-up phases. Parsley adds a mild flavor and a touch of vitamins, while the strained consistency keeps it light on the stomach.

Ingredients:

- 2 large carrots, chopped

- 2 celery stalks, chopped

- 1 small onion, quartered

- 1 small zucchini, chopped

- 1 handful fresh parsley, stems included

- 1 clove garlic, peeled and lightly crushed (optional)

- 6 cups water

- Salt to taste

Instructions:

1. In a large pot, combine carrots, celery, onion, zucchini, parsley, garlic (if using), and water.

2. Bring to a boil, then reduce the heat and let it simmer for 30–40 minutes, or until the vegetables are soft and the broth is flavorful.

3. Remove from heat and strain the broth through a fine mesh sieve, discarding the solids.

4. Add salt to taste and stir until dissolved.

Serving Suggestion: Pour the strained broth into a mug or bowl and sip slowly. This broth is hydrating, gentle, and provides light nourishment while helping to calm the digestive system.

Carrot and Ginger Soup (strained)

This Carrot and Ginger Soup is a warm, nourishing option that's gentle on the digestive system. The carrots provide essential nutrients, while ginger offers anti-inflammatory and soothing benefits. Straining the soup makes it even easier to digest, making it ideal for the flare-up phase of diverticulitis.

Ingredients:

- 4 large carrots, peeled and chopped

- 1 small potato, peeled and diced (optional, for a creamier texture)

- 1-inch piece of fresh ginger, peeled and sliced

- 4 cups low-sodium vegetable or chicken broth

- 1 tablespoon olive oil

- Salt to taste

- Fresh herbs (such as parsley or cilantro) for garnish (optional)

Instructions:

1. In a large pot, heat the olive oil over medium heat. Add the carrots, potato (if using), and ginger, and sauté for 3–5 minutes until slightly softened.

2. Add the broth, bring to a boil, then reduce the heat and let it simmer for 20–25 minutes, or until the vegetables are very soft.

3. Remove the pot from heat. Use an immersion blender or transfer the soup to a blender and puree until smooth.

4. Strain the soup through a fine mesh sieve or cheesecloth to remove any remaining solids, making it extra smooth and easy to digest.

5. Season with salt to taste and garnish with fresh herbs if desired.

Serving Suggestion: Serve warm in small sips to enjoy its soothing qualities. This strained carrot and ginger soup is an excellent choice for gentle nourishment, providing hydration and essential vitamins without stressing the digestive system.

Potato and Leek Puree (liquid consistency)

This Potato and Leek Puree is a comforting and mild dish that's easy on the digestive system. The potatoes provide a smooth texture, and leeks add a subtle, gentle flavor. Blending the soup to a liquid consistency makes it ideal for those experiencing a diverticulitis flare-up.

Ingredients:

- 2 medium potatoes, peeled and diced

- 1 small leek, white and light green parts only, cleaned and sliced

- 3 cups low-sodium vegetable or chicken broth

- 1 tablespoon olive oil or butter

- Salt to taste

- Fresh herbs (such as chives or parsley) for garnish (optional)

Instructions:

1. In a large pot, heat the olive oil or butter over medium heat. Add the sliced leek and sauté for 3–4 minutes until softened but not browned.

2. Add the diced potatoes and broth to the pot. Bring to a boil, then reduce the heat and let it simmer for 15–20 minutes, or until the potatoes are tender.

3. Remove the pot from heat. Use an immersion blender, or transfer the mixture to a blender, and puree until very smooth.

4. Add more broth or water as needed to reach a liquid, soup-like consistency.

5. Season with salt to taste, and garnish with fresh herbs if desired.

Serving Suggestion: Serve warm in a small bowl or mug. This potato and leek puree offers a gentle, nourishing option during flare-ups, providing smooth, easily digestible nutrition.

Smooth Blends and Juices

Smooth blends and juices can be refreshing, nutrient-rich options that are gentle on the digestive system, especially during sensitive periods or flare-ups. When prepared with carefully selected ingredients, they offer hydration, essential vitamins, and digestive support. Here are some recipes and tips for creating easy-to-digest blends that are both soothing and nourishing.

Benefits of Smooth Blends and Juices

1. Hydration: Juices and smoothies provide fluids that help keep the body hydrated, which is especially important during digestive flare-ups.

2. Easily Digestible Nutrients: Blending fruits and vegetables breaks down fibers, making it easier for the body to absorb nutrients.

3. Soothing Ingredients: Ingredients like ginger, cucumber, and coconut water can be particularly gentle and soothing to the digestive system.

Recipes

1. Coconut Water Smoothie with Papaya

Papaya is rich in enzymes like papain, which can aid digestion, while coconut water provides natural electrolytes for hydration.

Ingredients: Coconut water, diced fresh papaya, a small slice of banana for creaminess (optional).

Instructions: Blend all ingredients until smooth, adding more coconut water to reach desired consistency. Enjoy immediately.

2. Aloe Vera and Cucumber Juice

Aloe vera is known for its soothing properties, and cucumber adds hydration and a light, refreshing flavor.

Ingredients: Aloe vera gel (1-2 tablespoons), 1/2 cucumber (peeled and chopped), water, and a splash of lemon juice (optional).

Instructions: Blend the aloe vera, cucumber, and water until smooth. Strain if desired and drink fresh.

3. Apple-Ginger Digestive Blend

Apples are high in fiber (especially when peeled), and ginger helps reduce nausea and inflammation in the digestive tract.

Ingredients: 1 apple (peeled and sliced), 1/2 teaspoon fresh grated ginger, water, and honey (optional).

Instructions: Blend the apple and ginger with water until smooth. Strain if desired for a lighter juice, and add honey to taste.

4. Carrot and Apple Juice with Mint

Carrots and apples are both gentle on the stomach, and fresh mint adds a soothing, refreshing touch.

Ingredients: 1 carrot (peeled and chopped), 1 apple (peeled and sliced), a few fresh mint leaves, and water.

Instructions: Blend carrot, apple, mint, and water until smooth. Strain if preferred, and enjoy chilled.

Tips for Making Smooth Blends and Juices

- Strain if Needed: If fiber content is a concern, strain the blend to remove any remaining pulp.

- Use Fresh Ingredients: Fresh fruits and vegetables offer the best flavor and nutritional content.

- Avoid Added Sugars: Rely on natural sweetness from fruits rather than added sugars for optimal digestive health.

- Keep Ingredients Simple: Limiting each recipe to a few ingredients can help avoid any irritation from complex combinations.

Smooth blends and juices can be a gentle and revitalizing way to consume essential nutrients, keep hydrated, and support the digestive system in a manageable and soothing form.

Coconut Water Smoothie with Papaya

This Coconut Water Smoothie with Papaya is a light, hydrating drink that's gentle on the digestive system and perfect for a flare-up phase. Coconut water provides natural electrolytes, while papaya contains digestive enzymes that can aid in soothing the stomach.

Ingredients:

- 1 cup coconut water (unsweetened)

- 1/2 cup fresh or frozen papaya, diced

- 1/4 banana (optional, for added creaminess)

- 1 teaspoon honey or maple syrup (optional, for a touch of sweetness)

Instructions:

1. Place the coconut water, papaya, banana (if using), and honey or maple syrup (if using) into a blender.

2. Blend until smooth, ensuring there are no chunks left.

3. Pour into a glass and enjoy immediately.

Serving Suggestion: Enjoy this smoothie as a refreshing snack or light meal. The combination of hydrating coconut water and digestive-friendly papaya is ideal for soothing and nourishing your body during sensitive digestive phases.

Apple and Ginger Smoothie (strained)

This Apple and Ginger Smoothie is a soothing, slightly sweet drink with the digestive benefits of ginger and the fiber-rich properties of apple (even when strained). Straining makes it gentler on the stomach, creating a smooth, light consistency.

Ingredients:

- 1 medium apple, peeled and chopped

- 1/2 teaspoon fresh ginger, grated

- 1/2 cup water or coconut water (for added electrolytes)

- 1 teaspoon honey or maple syrup (optional, for extra sweetness)

Instructions:

1. Add the apple, ginger, and water or coconut water to a blender.

2. Blend until smooth, ensuring the apple and ginger are fully combined.

3. Strain the mixture through a fine mesh sieve to remove any pulp, creating a clear and gentle smoothie.

4. Pour into a glass, add honey or maple syrup if desired, and enjoy immediately.

Serving Suggestion: This strained smoothie is perfect for a light, digestive-friendly snack. The ginger adds a subtle zing while promoting digestive comfort, making it a suitable choice during flare-ups.

Clear Cucumber and Melon Juice

This Clear Cucumber and Melon Juice is a refreshing, hydrating drink that's gentle on the digestive system. Both cucumber and melon have a high water content, making this juice ideal for hydration during sensitive digestive periods. The mild flavors blend well together, resulting in a light, cooling beverage.

Ingredients:

- 1/2 cucumber, peeled and chopped

- 1 cup honeydew or cantaloupe melon, chopped

- 1/4 cup water (adjust as needed for desired consistency)

- Ice cubes (optional, for serving)

Instructions:

1. Place the cucumber, melon, and water in a blender. Blend until smooth and well combined.

2. Strain the mixture through a fine mesh sieve to remove pulp, resulting in a clear juice.

3. Pour into a glass, add ice cubes if desired, and enjoy immediately.

Serving Suggestion: Serve this juice chilled for a refreshing, hydrating drink that's gentle on the stomach. The combination of cucumber and melon makes it naturally sweet, hydrating, and soothing.

Chapter 3

Recovery Phase Recipes

The recovery phase is a crucial period for gently reintroducing nutrients while allowing the digestive system to heal. In this stage, it's important to focus on foods that provide essential nutrients, are easy to digest, and help reduce inflammation. These recipes include soft, mild ingredients and use preparation techniques like pureeing and steaming to ensure smooth textures and gentle digestion.

Goals for the Recovery Phase

1. Nourishment: Provide balanced nutrition with easily digestible proteins, healthy fats, and gentle carbohydrates to support healing.

2. Anti-Inflammatory Ingredients: Include foods like turmeric, ginger, and leafy greens, which may reduce inflammation in the gut.

3. Gradual Fiber Reintroduction: Slowly reintroduce fiber-rich foods in a manageable way, focusing on cooked and soft options that don't irritate the digestive system.

Recipes

1. Butternut Squash and Carrot Puree

This puree is rich in beta-carotene, gentle on digestion, and has a naturally sweet flavor that's comforting and nourishing.

Ingredients: Butternut squash, carrots, a pinch of salt, and a drizzle of olive oil.

Instructions: Steam or roast squash and carrots until tender, then blend with a bit of water or broth to reach a smooth consistency.

2. Mashed Sweet Potatoes with Olive Oil

Sweet potatoes are a fantastic source of fiber, vitamins, and minerals. Mashing them with olive oil keeps them smooth and easy on the stomach.

Ingredients: Sweet potatoes, olive oil, salt, and optional herbs like parsley.

Instructions: Boil sweet potatoes until tender, then mash with olive oil and salt. For extra smoothness, blend in a food processor.

3. Soft-Cooked Salmon with Steamed Spinach

Salmon is rich in omega-3 fatty acids, which support anti-inflammatory processes, while steamed spinach adds gentle fiber and iron.

Ingredients: Salmon fillet, spinach, a drizzle of lemon juice, and olive oil.

Instructions: Bake or steam the salmon until fully cooked, and steam the spinach until soft. Serve together with a drizzle of olive oil and lemon juice.

4. Rice Porridge with Bone Broth

Rice porridge is a soft, warming meal that's easy to digest. Cooking it in bone broth provides added protein and minerals beneficial for gut health.

Ingredients: White rice, bone broth, a pinch of salt, and herbs for flavor (optional).

Instructions: Simmer rice in bone broth until soft and thickened to a porridge consistency. Season lightly.

5. Banana and Oat Smoothie

Bananas and oats are gentle, easily digestible foods. This smoothie is a great choice for slowly reintroducing fiber without overwhelming the digestive system.

Ingredients: Ripe banana, oats (cooked or soaked), almond milk or water, and honey (optional).

Instructions: Blend banana and soaked oats with almond milk or water until smooth. Add honey for extra sweetness, if desired.

Tips for Recovery Phase Meals

Cook Vegetables Thoroughly: Soft, cooked vegetables are easier to digest than raw ones.

Use Healthy Fats: A small amount of olive oil or avocado oil can add smoothness and help the body absorb fat-soluble vitamins.

Portion Control: Start with small servings to avoid overloading the digestive system, gradually increasing as tolerated.

By focusing on nutrient-dense, gentle foods, the recovery phase can be a time to rebuild strength and give the digestive system a supportive environment for healing. These recipes prioritize softness, nutrition, and simplicity to promote comfort and sustained wellness.

Tips for reintroducing soft foods and avoiding fiber irritants

Reintroducing soft foods after a diverticulitis flare-up requires a gentle, gradual approach to avoid irritating the digestive system. Start with low-fiber, easily digestible options such as mashed potatoes, bananas, applesauce, white rice, and well-cooked vegetables. These foods are gentle on the stomach, allowing it to heal while still providing essential nutrients. Proteins that are soft, like scrambled eggs, tofu, and tender fish, are also beneficial during this phase.

To make vegetables even easier to digest, try steaming or boiling them until they are very soft, breaking down the fibers that can otherwise be tough on the gut. Pureeing or mashing these foods further smooths their texture, reducing the likelihood of irritation. As you progress, consider incorporating foods with soluble fiber, like oatmeal or sweet potatoes, which are gentler than insoluble fiber options.

It's wise to avoid fiber-rich foods that are difficult to digest, such as raw vegetables, nuts, seeds, and popcorn, as these can be hard on a recovering digestive system. Peeling fruits and vegetables can help reduce fiber content, making them easier to tolerate. Whole grains may also be difficult initially, so refined grains like white rice can be a gentler choice.

Staying hydrated is important for digestion, especially as you slowly reintroduce fiber. Drinking water throughout the day and incorporating hydrating foods like cucumber, melon, and broth-based soups can further support your recovery. Adjusting your diet slowly and monitoring your comfort level helps create a smooth, irritation-free transition back to regular eating, supporting long-term digestive health and healing.

Simple and Soothing Breakfasts

Starting the day with a gentle, nourishing breakfast can be especially beneficial during diverticulitis recovery. Simple, easy-to-digest foods help ease the digestive system into the day, providing comfort and energy without irritation.

One option is warm oatmeal made with water or almond milk, cooked until very soft. Adding a drizzle of honey or a pinch of cinnamon enhances the flavor without overwhelming the stomach. Another soothing choice is a smooth banana smoothie, blending ripe banana with a bit of water or coconut milk until creamy. This smoothie provides potassium and natural sweetness that's easy on digestion.

Scrambled eggs or a soft-boiled egg can offer a gentle protein boost. Eggs are easy to digest and provide essential nutrients to start the day. For a bit of variety, try a dollop of applesauce on the side, which is low in fiber when strained and offers a mild sweetness.

For a warming breakfast, mashed sweet potatoes with a little olive oil or butter are filling, nutrient-dense, and gentle on the stomach. Cook the sweet potato until it's very soft, then mash it thoroughly for a comforting texture.

These simple, soothing breakfasts are not only gentle on the digestive system but also packed with essential nutrients to support healing and energy throughout the morning. Each option is adaptable to your needs, allowing for flexibility and comfort as you gradually reintroduce more foods.

Creamy Oatmeal with Banana and Honey (strained, optional))

This creamy oatmeal recipe provides a warm, gentle start to your day with soothing ingredients that are easy to digest. Bananas add natural sweetness and potassium, while a drizzle of honey enhances flavor. Straining the oatmeal is an optional step to achieve an even smoother texture if needed.

Ingredients:

- 1/2 cup rolled oats (or instant oats for softer texture)

- 1 cup water or almond milk

- 1/2 ripe banana, mashed

- 1 tsp honey (optional)

- A pinch of cinnamon (optional)

Instructions:

1. In a small saucepan, bring the water or almond milk to a gentle boil.

2. Stir in the oats and reduce the heat to low, allowing them to simmer until they become soft and creamy (about 5-10 minutes for rolled oats; 2-3 minutes for instant oats).

3. Once the oatmeal reaches your desired consistency, stir in the mashed banana for natural sweetness and creaminess.

4. If desired, strain the oatmeal through a fine mesh strainer to remove any larger particles for an even smoother texture.

5. Drizzle with honey and sprinkle with a pinch of cinnamon, if using, and serve warm.

This oatmeal is comforting and nutrient-rich, providing a soothing and easy-to-digest breakfast. Perfect for mornings when you want something nourishing yet gentle on your stomach.

Soft-Boiled Egg with Steamed Spinach

This simple breakfast combines protein and iron-rich spinach, offering a gentle yet nourishing option for sensitive digestion. Soft-boiled eggs are easy to digest, and steaming the spinach keeps it tender and mild.

Ingredients:

- 1 large egg

- 1/2 cup fresh spinach, rinsed

- A pinch of salt (optional)

- A drizzle of olive oil or a small pat of butter (optional)

Instructions:

1. Soft-Boil the Egg: Bring a small pot of water to a gentle boil. Carefully add the egg and cook for 5-6 minutes for a soft, creamy center. Once cooked, remove the egg and place it in a bowl of cold water to cool slightly, then peel.

2. Steam the Spinach: While the egg is cooking, place the spinach in a steamer or a heat-safe bowl over a pot of boiling water. Cover and steam for 2-3 minutes, until wilted and tender. Remove and season with a pinch of salt or a drizzle of olive oil, if desired.

3. Serve: Place the peeled soft-boiled egg on a plate with the steamed spinach on the side.

This dish is gentle, warm, and rich in essential nutrients to start your day. The tender spinach and creamy egg are both easy on the stomach, making it a great choice for digestive health.

Smooth Rice Porridge with Coconut Milk

This smooth and creamy rice porridge is a comforting, easy-to-digest breakfast option that's perfect for sensitive stomachs. Coconut milk adds a subtle richness and natural sweetness without overwhelming the digestive system.

Ingredients:

- 1/2 cup white rice (jasmine or basmati works well)

- 2 cups water

- 1/2 cup coconut milk (canned or carton)

- A pinch of salt

Optional toppings: drizzle of honey or maple syrup, a sprinkle of cinnamon, or a few soft slices of ripe banana

Instructions:

1. Cook the Rice: In a medium saucepan, combine the rice and water. Bring to a boil, then reduce the heat to low and cover. Simmer for 15-20 minutes, or until the rice is very soft and most of the water has been absorbed.

2. Blend the Porridge: Once the rice is cooked, add the coconut milk and a pinch of salt. Stir well and simmer for another 5 minutes, until the mixture

becomes creamy. For an even smoother texture, blend with an immersion blender or transfer to a regular blender and blend until smooth.

3. Serve: Pour the rice porridge into a bowl and add any desired toppings, such as a drizzle of honey or a few slices of banana, for added flavor and a touch of sweetness.

This gentle rice porridge is soothing and filling, with a mild coconut flavor that enhances its creamy texture. Perfect for mornings when you want a warm, comforting meal that's easy on the stomach.

Gentle Lunches

Gentle lunches are an ideal way to nourish yourself in the middle of the day without overloading your digestive system. These meals focus on soft, easy-to-digest ingredients that provide essential nutrients while remaining soothing and mild.

For those managing digestive sensitivity, think of meals that incorporate soft grains, pureed or steamed vegetables, and tender proteins. Soft-cooked grains like white rice, quinoa, or couscous can be paired with steamed or pureed vegetables, such as carrots, sweet potatoes, or zucchini. These vegetables offer vitamins and minerals in a form that's easy on the stomach.

For protein, tender options like shredded chicken, soft tofu, or poached fish are gentle choices that still offer filling, high-quality protein. Soft-cooked eggs, as in an egg drop soup or egg salad, can also make a satisfying, protein-rich addition.

Soups and stews are perfect for gentle lunches, especially when made with a base of clear broth and easy-to-digest ingredients. Pureed soups, such as carrot and ginger, or zucchini and potato, provide warmth and nourishment without being heavy. Straining the soup can also help reduce any fibrous content, making it even easier on digestion.

These gentle lunch ideas offer a balance of essential nutrients, helping to sustain energy and promote healing, all while respecting the needs of a sensitive digestive system.

Scrambled Eggs with Fresh Herbs

This simple, gentle dish is packed with protein and flavor, making it an excellent choice for a soothing, easy-to-digest lunch or breakfast. Fresh herbs add a hint of flavor without overpowering the stomach, and the soft texture of scrambled eggs is ideal for sensitive digestion.

Ingredients:

- 2 large eggs

- 1 tablespoon milk or water

- Salt (optional)

- Fresh herbs (such as parsley, chives, or basil), finely chopped

- 1 teaspoon olive oil or butter

Instructions:

1. Prepare the Eggs: In a small bowl, whisk the eggs with milk or water until smooth. Add a pinch of salt, if desired.

2. Cook the Eggs: In a nonstick skillet, heat the olive oil or butter over low to medium heat. Pour in the egg mixture.

3. Scramble Gently: Using a spatula, stir the eggs slowly and continuously as they cook, keeping the heat low to avoid overcooking. Cook until the eggs are soft and creamy.

4. Add Herbs: Once the eggs are nearly done, sprinkle in the fresh herbs and stir gently to combine.

5. Serve Warm: Transfer to a plate and enjoy warm.

These soft, flavorful scrambled eggs are light, nourishing, and easy on the stomach—perfect for a gentle, satisfying meal that won't disrupt digestion.

Soft Mashed Sweet Potatoes with Olive Oil

This dish combines the natural sweetness of tender, mashed sweet potatoes with the smooth richness of olive oil. It's a comforting, nutrient-rich option that's gentle on the stomach and perfect for a soothing lunch or side dish.

Ingredients:

- 1 medium sweet potato

- 1-2 teaspoons olive oil

- Salt (optional)

- Fresh herbs, like parsley or chives, for garnish (optional)

Instructions:

1. Cook the Sweet Potato: Peel and chop the sweet potato into cubes for faster cooking. In a medium pot, bring water to a boil and add the sweet potato. Boil for 10-15 minutes or until very soft.

2. Mash: Drain the sweet potato and transfer it to a bowl. Add the olive oil and mash with a fork or potato masher until smooth and creamy. Add a small pinch of salt if desired.

3. Serve Warm: For a garnish, sprinkle with a small amount of finely chopped fresh herbs if your stomach tolerates them.

This creamy mashed sweet potato dish is easy to digest and packed with nutrients, offering a gentle, soothing meal option for anyone with a sensitive stomach.

Poached Chicken with Pureed Carrots and Zucchini

Poached Chicken with Pureed Carrots and Zucchini

This gentle, nutrient-dense meal combines tender poached chicken with smooth pureed carrots and zucchini, making it an ideal choice for sensitive digestion. The soft textures and mild flavors offer a soothing and nourishing lunch option.

Ingredients:

1 small chicken breast (boneless and skinless)

Salt (optional)

1 small carrot, peeled and chopped

1/2 small zucchini, chopped

1 teaspoon olive oil or a small pat of butter (optional)

Instructions:

1. Poach the Chicken: In a small pot, add the chicken breast and cover with water. Bring to a gentle simmer over medium heat. Lower the heat, cover, and poach the chicken for 12-15 minutes or

until it's fully cooked and tender. Remove the chicken and let it rest before slicing or shredding it into bite-sized pieces.

2. Cook the Vegetables: While the chicken is cooking, add the chopped carrot and zucchini to a separate pot with enough water to cover. Simmer for 10-12 minutes or until very soft.

3. Puree the Vegetables: Drain the vegetables and transfer them to a blender or food processor. Add the olive oil or butter for extra smoothness, then blend until you achieve a creamy puree. Add a small pinch of salt if desired.

4. Serve: Plate the poached chicken alongside the carrot and zucchini puree.

This mild, easy-to-digest meal provides a balanced mix of protein and vegetables, ideal for anyone needing a gentle yet nutritious option.

Light Dinners

Light dinners are a great way to end the day on a gentle, satisfying note without overwhelming your digestive system. When managing a sensitive stomach, it's beneficial to focus on meals that are easy to digest, nutrient-dense, and low in heavy spices or rich sauces. Light dinners emphasize gentle ingredients like steamed or pureed vegetables, lean proteins, and soft grains, all prepared in ways that enhance digestibility and flavor.

Soups, broths, and soft-cooked dishes like baked fish or tender chicken are excellent choices. These options provide protein and essential nutrients without being too filling or difficult to digest. For example, poached or steamed white fish served with pureed vegetables, such as mashed carrots or steamed zucchini, offers both nourishment and a soothing texture.

Other gentle dinner ideas include soft-cooked grains like quinoa or rice paired with steamed vegetables and mild seasonings. Adding a drizzle of olive oil or a light broth can enhance flavor without adding heaviness. Light vegetable stews or blended soups made with ingredients like butternut squash, sweet potatoes, or leeks are warming and nutrient-rich, providing a comforting end to the day.

These light dinner options are perfect for those aiming to manage digestive discomfort while still enjoying balanced, wholesome meals. They support restful digestion and help prepare the body for a good night's sleep.

Baked Cod with Mashed Potatoes

This simple, gentle dish pairs tender baked cod with creamy mashed potatoes for a soothing, light dinner that's easy on the stomach. Cod is a mild, lean fish that's packed with protein and essential nutrients, while the soft mashed potatoes provide comfort and energy without overwhelming the digestive system.

Ingredients:

- 1 cod fillet (about 4-6 oz)

- 1 teaspoon olive oil

- Salt and pepper (optional, for taste)

- Fresh herbs, such as parsley or dill, for garnish (optional)

For the Mashed Potatoes:

- 1 medium potato, peeled and cubed

- 1-2 teaspoons olive oil or a small pat of butter

- Salt (optional)

Instructions:

1. Prepare the Cod: Preheat your oven to 375°F (190°C). Place the cod fillet on a baking sheet lined with parchment paper or lightly greased with olive oil. Drizzle a teaspoon of olive oil over the fish and season lightly with salt and pepper if desired. Bake for 12-15 minutes, or until the fish is opaque and flakes easily with a fork.

2. Cook the Potatoes: While the fish is baking, add the cubed potatoes to a pot of water. Bring to a boil,

then simmer for 10-12 minutes, or until the potatoes are very soft. Drain well.

3. Mash the Potatoes: Transfer the potatoes to a bowl. Add olive oil or butter and a pinch of salt if desired, then mash until smooth and creamy.

4. Serve: Plate the baked cod alongside the mashed potatoes. Garnish with a sprinkle of fresh herbs if desired.

This light, nourishing meal is gentle yet flavorful, making it a great option for dinner when you want something satisfying and easy on the stomach.

Steamed and Mashed Cauliflower with a Touch of Garlic

This mashed cauliflower is a lighter, low-carb alternative to mashed potatoes, with a smooth, creamy texture and a hint of garlic for subtle flavor. Cauliflower is easy to digest and gentle on the stomach, making this dish an excellent side for those seeking comfort without heaviness.

Ingredients:

- 1 medium head of cauliflower, cut into florets

- 1 clove garlic, peeled (optional)

- 1-2 teaspoons olive oil or a small pat of butter

- Salt (optional)

- Fresh herbs, like chives or parsley, for garnish (optional)

Instructions:

1. Steam the Cauliflower: In a steamer basket over boiling water, add the cauliflower florets and garlic clove (if using). Cover and steam for about 10-12 minutes, or until the cauliflower is very soft.

2. Mash the Cauliflower: Drain the steamed cauliflower and transfer it to a food processor or

blender. Add olive oil or butter, and a pinch of salt if desired. Blend until smooth and creamy. If needed, add a tablespoon of warm water to reach a creamier consistency.

3. Serve: Scoop the mashed cauliflower into a serving dish and garnish with finely chopped herbs if desired.

This mashed cauliflower with a touch of garlic is light yet satisfying, offering a warm, comforting side that pairs well with a variety of main dishes and supports easy digestion.

Soft Polenta with Stewed Mushrooms (strained)

This soft polenta with delicate stewed mushrooms offers a creamy, comforting dish that's gentle on the digestive system. Polenta provides a smooth, easily digestible base, while the mushrooms add earthy flavor. Straining the mushroom mixture ensures only the smoothest consistency for sensitive stomachs.

Ingredients:

- 1/2 cup polenta or cornmeal

- 2 cups water or low-sodium vegetable broth

- 1 teaspoon olive oil or butter

- Salt (optional)

For the Stewed Mushrooms:

- 1/2 cup mushrooms, thinly sliced (such as button or cremini)

- 1/4 cup water or low-sodium vegetable broth

- 1 small clove garlic, peeled (optional)

- Salt (optional)

Instructions:

1. Cook the Polenta: In a pot, bring water or broth to a boil. Slowly whisk in the polenta, reducing the heat to low. Stir frequently to prevent lumps,

cooking for 15-20 minutes or until creamy. Add olive oil or butter and a pinch of salt if desired.

2. Stew the Mushrooms: In a separate pan, add mushrooms, water or broth, and garlic (if using). Simmer on low heat for 10-12 minutes until the mushrooms are soft and tender.

3. Strain the Mushrooms: Once the mushrooms are stewed, remove the garlic if used, then strain the mushrooms, reserving the liquid to drizzle over the polenta.

4. Serve: Spoon the creamy polenta into a bowl, topping with the strained mushrooms and a drizzle of the reserved liquid for extra flavor.

This dish provides a warm, smooth, and soothing meal that's rich in gentle flavors and easy on the stomach.

Snacks and Small Bites

When managing digestive health, snacks and small bites can be a great way to keep energy up without overwhelming the stomach. Ideal snacks for sensitive digestion are light, easy to chew, and nutrient-dense, with a focus on gentle ingredients that won't irritate the digestive tract. In this section, you'll find snack options that are not only comforting but also supportive of digestive health.

Soft fruits, like bananas or applesauce, are perfect for a quick energy boost and provide natural fiber that's gentle and easy to digest. Blended or mashed snacks, such as a smooth avocado spread or a small serving of creamy yogurt (if dairy is tolerated), offer healthy fats and probiotics that may benefit gut health. Nut butters, especially in small amounts and perhaps on a mild rice cracker, provide protein and healthy fats while being gentle on the stomach.

Gentle, homemade options like steamed veggie sticks, small servings of mashed sweet potato, or rice cakes with a thin layer of almond or peanut butter make for convenient and satisfying snacks.

These choices allow you to nourish your body throughout the day, even during recovery phases.

Each of these snack ideas is crafted with comfort in mind, helping to keep your digestive system at ease while satisfying hunger between meals.

Applesauce with Cinnamon

This simple and soothing applesauce with a hint of cinnamon makes a comforting snack that's easy on the stomach. Apples are gentle on the digestive system when cooked, and the cinnamon adds a touch of warmth and flavor without adding any heaviness.

Ingredients:

- 2 medium apples, peeled, cored, and chopped (such as Gala or Fuji)

- 1/4 cup water

- 1/4 teaspoon ground cinnamon (optional)

- A dash of honey or maple syrup (optional, for extra sweetness)

Instructions:

1. Cook the Apples: In a small saucepan, combine the chopped apples and water. Cover and cook over medium-low heat for 10-15 minutes, or until the apples are very soft.

2. Mash or Blend: Once the apples are soft, mash them with a fork for a chunky texture or blend for a smoother consistency. Stir in the cinnamon and honey or maple syrup if desired.

3. Serve: Allow the applesauce to cool slightly before eating. Enjoy it warm or chilled as a gentle, naturally sweet snack.

This homemade applesauce is gentle, lightly spiced, and ideal for a sensitive stomach, providing both comfort and a bit of natural sweetness.

Pear and Banana Puree

This creamy pear and banana puree is a naturally sweet and soothing snack that's easy to digest. Both pears and bananas are gentle on the stomach and provide essential vitamins and fiber in a form that's easy to absorb. The smooth texture makes it an excellent option for those recovering from digestive discomfort.

Ingredients:

- 1 ripe pear, peeled, cored, and chopped

- 1 ripe banana, peeled

- 1/4 cup water (or as needed for desired consistency)

- A pinch of cinnamon (optional)

Instructions:

1. Prepare the Fruit: In a small saucepan, add the chopped pear and a little water. Cook over low heat for about 5-7 minutes, or until the pear is soft.

2. Blend the Fruit: Once the pear is soft, add the banana and the cooked pear to a blender or food processor. Blend until smooth, adding more water if needed to achieve a smooth, puree consistency.

3. Serve: Optionally, sprinkle a pinch of cinnamon for extra flavor. Serve immediately or store in the refrigerator for later.

This pear and banana puree is a gentle, nutritious, and delicious snack that's perfect for anyone seeking a light bite that's easy on the digestive system.

Soft Rice Pudding with Almond Milk

This soft rice pudding made with almond milk is a comforting and easy-to-digest snack. It's naturally dairy-free, making it suitable for those who are lactose intolerant or prefer plant-based options. The creamy texture of almond milk combined with the soft rice creates a gentle and soothing treat, ideal for sensitive stomachs.

Ingredients:

- 1/2 cup white rice (short-grain works best for creaminess)

- 2 cups unsweetened almond milk

- 1-2 tablespoons honey or maple syrup (optional)

- 1/4 teaspoon ground cinnamon (optional)

- 1 teaspoon vanilla extract (optional)

- Pinch of salt

Instructions:

1. Cook the Rice: In a medium saucepan, add the rice, almond milk, and a pinch of salt. Bring the

mixture to a simmer over medium heat, stirring occasionally.

2. Simmer: Once it reaches a simmer, reduce the heat to low and cover the saucepan. Cook for 25-30 minutes, stirring occasionally to prevent sticking. If the pudding gets too thick, add a little more almond milk as needed to reach a creamy consistency.

3. Sweeten and Flavor: Once the rice is tender and the pudding has thickened, stir in the honey or maple syrup for sweetness, along with cinnamon and vanilla extract if using. Let it cook for an additional 5-10 minutes to allow the flavors to meld.

4. Serve: Allow the rice pudding to cool slightly before serving. It can be enjoyed warm or chilled, depending on your preference.

This rice pudding is a soothing, naturally sweet dessert or snack that's easy on the stomach and provides a gentle, comforting option for digestive health.

Chapter 4

Maintenance Phase Recipes (High-Fiber and Anti-Inflammatory Diets)

As you progress from the flare-up and recovery phases, it's important to focus on maintaining long-term digestive health. The maintenance phase emphasizes incorporating high-fiber and anti-inflammatory foods that support gut healing, prevent future flare-ups, and reduce inflammation. This stage is about transitioning from easily digestible foods to meals that nourish your digestive system, promote regularity, and foster overall well-being.

A high-fiber diet is crucial for long-term digestive health. Fiber promotes regular bowel movements, helps control blood sugar levels, and aids in managing cholesterol. Incorporating fiber-rich foods such as whole grains, legumes, fruits, and vegetables is key to a healthy diet in the maintenance phase. However, it's important to introduce fiber gradually and be mindful of individual tolerance levels, as too much fiber too quickly can irritate the digestive tract.

Anti-inflammatory foods are equally important, as they help soothe the gut and prevent inflammation that may lead to flare-ups. These include foods rich in omega-3 fatty acids (such as flaxseeds, chia seeds, and salmon), antioxidants (found in colorful fruits and vegetables), and herbs and spices like turmeric and ginger, which have natural anti-inflammatory properties.

In this chapter, you will find recipes that focus on these healing nutrients, providing a balance of flavors and textures that are both satisfying and gentle on the stomach. From hearty salads and grain bowls to anti-inflammatory smoothies and soups, these recipes will help you build a diverse and nutrient-dense diet that supports your digestive health in the long term. With a focus on balance and nourishment, these meals can become part of your everyday routine as you maintain a healthy and resilient gut.

Importance of fiber and anti-inflammatory foods for long-term health

Fiber and anti-inflammatory foods play a key role in supporting long-term health, especially for individuals managing digestive conditions like diverticulitis. Fiber, found in fruits, vegetables, whole grains, and legumes, is essential for promoting regular bowel movements and preventing constipation, which reduces pressure on the colon and minimizes the risk of flare-ups. Soluble fiber, in particular, dissolves in water to form a gel-like substance that aids in slowing digestion and promoting better nutrient absorption. Insoluble fiber adds bulk to the stool, helping it pass more easily, which can be beneficial for overall gut health.

Anti-inflammatory foods are equally important, as chronic inflammation can contribute to a range of digestive and systemic health issues. Foods rich in omega-3 fatty acids, like flaxseeds and fatty fish, as well as those high in antioxidants, such as berries and leafy greens, help reduce inflammation in the body. Anti-inflammatory spices, including turmeric and ginger, have been shown to calm the digestive tract, reducing the likelihood of discomfort and flare-ups.

Including a balanced mix of fiber and anti-inflammatory foods in your diet can help maintain a healthy gut, support immune function, and reduce the risk of chronic diseases. Together, these foods create a solid foundation for long-term health by improving digestive resilience and fostering an environment that supports healing and overall well-being.

Energizing Breakfasts

A nutritious breakfast sets the tone for the day, providing essential energy, focus, and nutrients to fuel your body. For those managing digestive health, it's important to start the day with meals that are both gentle on the stomach and packed with fiber, protein, and anti-inflammatory ingredients. Energizing breakfasts can help stabilize blood sugar, reduce inflammation, and promote a steady release of energy throughout the morning, which is essential for maintaining digestive comfort and overall wellness.

In this chapter, you'll find breakfast recipes designed to energize you without overwhelming your digestive system. Each recipe incorporates foods that are easy to digest while also providing important nutrients like vitamins, minerals, and fiber. You'll see options like overnight oats topped with soothing berries, creamy smoothies packed with anti-inflammatory fruits and greens, and egg-based dishes that supply protein without being too heavy.

These breakfasts emphasize balance, combining sources of healthy carbs, protein, and fats that will keep you feeling full and energized. Incorporating these recipes into your morning routine can help you approach each day with the energy and resilience needed to support both your digestive health and overall well-being.

Overnight Oats with Steamed Berries

This simple and delicious overnight oats recipe is high in fiber and gentle on digestion. Oats provide soluble fiber, which helps promote gut health, while steaming the berries makes them easier to digest and reduces acidity. This recipe is perfect for a nourishing breakfast that supports digestive wellness.

Ingredients:

- 1/2 cup rolled oats

- 1/2 cup almond milk (or your preferred milk)

- 1/4 cup water

- 1/2 teaspoon chia seeds (optional for extra fiber)

- 1/2 cup mixed berries (blueberries, strawberries, or raspberries)

- 1/4 teaspoon honey or maple syrup (optional for sweetness)

- A pinch of cinnamon (optional)

Instructions:

1. Prepare the Oats: In a jar or bowl, combine the oats, almond milk, water, and chia seeds (if using).

117

Stir well to ensure the oats are fully coated. Cover and refrigerate overnight, or for at least 4 hours.

2. Steam the Berries: In a small saucepan, add the berries with a tablespoon of water. Cover and steam over low heat for about 5 minutes, or until the berries are softened. Mash slightly with a fork for a jam-like consistency.

3. Assemble: In the morning, give the oats a quick stir and top them with the steamed berries. Drizzle with honey or maple syrup and sprinkle with cinnamon if desired.

4. Serve: Enjoy the oats chilled straight from the fridge, or warm them slightly if you prefer.

This overnight oats recipe with steamed berries is a fiber-rich, soothing breakfast that's perfect for maintaining digestive health while adding a burst of flavor and natural sweetness.

Greek Yogurt with Honey and Softened Pear

This simple and soothing breakfast combines the probiotic benefits of Greek yogurt with the natural sweetness of honey and the gentle texture of softened pear. Greek yogurt provides protein and beneficial bacteria that support gut health, while pears offer fiber that's easy on digestion, especially when softened.

Ingredients:

- 1 cup plain Greek yogurt

- 1 ripe pear, peeled and chopped

- 1 tablespoon honey (or to taste)

- 1/4 teaspoon cinnamon (optional)

Instructions:

1. Soften the Pear: Place the chopped pear in a small saucepan with a splash of water. Cover and cook over low heat for 5-7 minutes, or until the pear

is soft and tender. Remove from heat and let it cool slightly.

2. Assemble: Spoon the Greek yogurt into a bowl and top with the softened pear pieces.

3. Add Honey and Cinnamon: Drizzle honey over the yogurt and pear, and sprinkle with cinnamon if desired.

4. Serve: Enjoy immediately as a light, refreshing breakfast or snack.

This Greek yogurt with honey and softened pear offers a creamy, lightly sweetened start to your day that's gentle on the stomach and rich in nutrients to support energy and digestion.

Flaxseed and Berry Smoothie

This delicious smoothie combines fiber-rich flaxseeds with antioxidant-packed berries for a refreshing and nutritious start to your day. Flaxseeds provide omega-3 fatty acids and soluble fiber, which support digestive health, while berries bring anti-inflammatory benefits that can help reduce irritation in the digestive tract.

Ingredients:

- 1/2 cup mixed berries (blueberries, strawberries, raspberries; fresh or frozen)

- 1 tablespoon ground flaxseeds

- 1/2 banana (optional for added creaminess)

- 3/4 cup almond milk (or your preferred milk)

- 1/4 cup Greek yogurt (optional for extra protein)

- 1/4 teaspoon honey or maple syrup (optional for added sweetness)

- A few ice cubes (optional for a thicker texture)

Instructions:

1. Blend Ingredients: In a blender, combine the mixed berries, ground flaxseeds, banana, almond milk, Greek yogurt, and honey or maple syrup. Add a few ice cubes if you prefer a thicker smoothie.

2. Blend Until Smooth: Blend on high until all ingredients are fully combined and the smoothie reaches a smooth, creamy consistency.

3. Serve: Pour into a glass and enjoy immediately.

This flaxseed and berry smoothie is a nutritious, energizing option that's packed with fiber, antioxidants, and healthy fats to keep you full, promote digestive health, and support inflammation reduction throughout the day.

Fiber-Friendly Lunches

Fiber-friendly lunches can be satisfying and nourishing, while also gentle on the digestive system, especially for those managing conditions like diverticulitis. These meals emphasize foods rich in soluble fiber, which helps ease digestion, stabilize blood sugar, and promote steady energy. Including moderate amounts of fiber in lunch helps you feel full longer, keeps digestion smooth, and supports overall gut health.

A fiber-friendly lunch can include ingredients like soft-cooked vegetables, lean proteins, and gentle whole grains. For example, dishes like a quinoa and steamed vegetable bowl offer a hearty mix of fiber, protein, and essential nutrients while being easy on the stomach. Soft-cooked carrots, zucchini, and bell peppers pair well with quinoa, which is a great source of plant-based protein and fiber.

For those who enjoy wraps or sandwiches, a whole-grain wrap filled with mashed avocado, soft lettuce, and a light protein like poached chicken or scrambled egg can offer balanced fiber without being too heavy. Adding a spread of hummus can also provide both flavor and an extra boost of fiber.

Another great option is a hearty vegetable soup with lentils, which provides protein and soluble fiber, promoting satiety and gut health without overloading the digestive system.

These fiber-friendly lunch options not only support a healthy gut but also help maintain stable energy and blood sugar levels throughout the afternoon, making them a great choice for both digestive wellness and overall health.

Lentil and Vegetable Soup with Turmeric

This comforting lentil and vegetable soup is packed with fiber, protein, and anti-inflammatory ingredients, making it a perfect option for a fiber-friendly lunch. The lentils provide a solid source of soluble fiber, which is great for digestion, while the turmeric adds anti-inflammatory benefits to help soothe the digestive system. The vegetables give the soup additional nutrients and fiber, promoting overall gut health.

Ingredients:

- 1 cup dry lentils, rinsed

- 1 tablespoon olive oil

- 1 small onion, chopped

- 2 garlic cloves, minced

- 2 carrots, peeled and diced

- 1 zucchini, diced

- 1 small potato, peeled and cubed

- 1 teaspoon ground turmeric

- 1/2 teaspoon ground cumin (optional)

- 4 cups vegetable broth (low-sodium)

- Salt and pepper, to taste

- Fresh parsley for garnish (optional)

Instructions:

1. Prepare Vegetables: In a large pot, heat olive oil over medium heat. Add the chopped onion and

garlic and sauté for 2-3 minutes, until fragrant and softened.

2. Cook Vegetables: Add the diced carrots, zucchini, and potato to the pot. Stir to combine, then cook for another 5 minutes, allowing the vegetables to soften slightly.

3. Add Lentils and Spices: Stir in the rinsed lentils, turmeric, and cumin (if using). Cook for 1-2 minutes to allow the spices to toast.

4. Simmer: Pour in the vegetable broth and bring the soup to a boil. Once boiling, reduce the heat to low and let it simmer for 30-40 minutes, or until the lentils and vegetables are tender. Stir occasionally and check the soup's consistency; if it's too thick, add more broth or water as needed.

5. Season: Season with salt and pepper to taste.

6. Serve: Ladle the soup into bowls and garnish with fresh parsley if desired. Serve warm.

This lentil and vegetable soup with turmeric is a soothing, nourishing meal that's rich in fiber and anti-inflammatory properties. It's perfect for those looking to support digestive health while enjoying a hearty, flavorful meal.

Quinoa and Roasted Vegetable Bowl

This vibrant quinoa and roasted vegetable bowl is a fiber-packed meal, offering a perfect balance of plant-based protein, healthy fats, and nutrient-rich vegetables. The quinoa provides both soluble and insoluble fiber, supporting digestion, while the roasted vegetables add vitamins, minerals, and an extra dose of fiber. The dish is lightly seasoned, making it easy on the stomach and perfect for those looking for a fiber-friendly, anti-inflammatory meal.

Ingredients:

- 1 cup quinoa (rinsed)

- 2 tablespoons olive oil

- 1 small sweet potato, peeled and diced

- 1 zucchini, sliced

- 1 bell pepper, chopped

- 1 small red onion, sliced

- 1 teaspoon ground cumin

- 1/2 teaspoon ground turmeric

- Salt and pepper to taste

- 1 tablespoon fresh parsley, chopped (optional)

- Lemon wedges for serving (optional)

Instructions:

1. Cook Quinoa: In a medium pot, combine the rinsed quinoa with 2 cups of water. Bring to a boil, then reduce the heat to low, cover, and simmer for

15-20 minutes, or until the quinoa is cooked and fluffy. Set aside.

2. Roast Vegetables: Preheat your oven to 400°F (200°C). In a bowl, toss the sweet potato, zucchini, bell pepper, and red onion with olive oil, cumin, turmeric, salt, and pepper. Spread the vegetables evenly on a baking sheet lined with parchment paper.

3. Roast: Roast the vegetables for 25-30 minutes, flipping halfway through, until they are tender and lightly browned.

4. Assemble the Bowl: Once the quinoa and vegetables are ready, assemble the bowl by placing a scoop of quinoa at the base. Top with the roasted vegetables.

5. Serve: Garnish with fresh parsley and serve with lemon wedges for a burst of citrus if desired.

This quinoa and roasted vegetable bowl is a nourishing, fiber-rich dish that supports digestive health and is easy to customize with your favorite vegetables. It's a satisfying, wholesome meal ideal for any time of day, offering both flavor and gut-friendly benefits.

Salmon Salad with Soft Lettuce and Olive Oil Dressing

This simple and nutrient-packed salmon salad is an ideal choice for those looking to support their digestive health while enjoying a light, satisfying meal. With omega-3-rich salmon, fiber from the soft lettuce, and healthy fats from the olive oil dressing, this dish is not only easy to digest but also anti-inflammatory, making it perfect for those in recovery or maintenance phases of digestive health.

Ingredients:

- 1 can of wild-caught salmon (or 1 cooked salmon fillet, flaked)

- 2 cups soft lettuce (such as butter lettuce, arugula, or baby spinach)

- 1/2 cucumber, thinly sliced

- 1/4 cup cherry tomatoes, halved

- 1/4 avocado, sliced (optional)

- 1 tablespoon olive oil

- 1 teaspoon lemon juice (or apple cider vinegar)

- Salt and pepper to taste

- Fresh herbs (such as dill or parsley) for garnish (optional)

Instructions:

1. Prepare the Salad: In a large bowl, place the soft lettuce leaves. Add the sliced cucumber, cherry tomatoes, and avocado (if using). Gently toss the ingredients together.

2. Flake the Salmon: If using canned salmon, drain it and flake it into large chunks. If you're using a cooked salmon fillet, flake it with a fork. Add the salmon on top of the salad.

3. Make the Dressing: In a small bowl, whisk together the olive oil, lemon juice (or apple cider vinegar), salt, and pepper to taste.

4. Assemble the Salad: Pour the dressing over the salad and toss gently to combine all ingredients. Garnish with fresh herbs like dill or parsley for extra flavor.

5. Serve: Enjoy immediately as a light, healthy lunch or dinner.

This salmon salad with soft lettuce and olive oil dressing is a nourishing, easy-to-digest meal that provides omega-3s, fiber, and anti-inflammatory properties, making it an excellent choice for those managing digestive issues while focusing on long-term gut health.

Hearty Dinners

Hearty dinners can play a crucial role in supporting digestive health while still providing satisfaction and nourishment. As individuals transition through the recovery or maintenance phases of diverticulitis, it's important to focus on meals that are rich in fiber, lean proteins, and essential nutrients but gentle on the digestive system. These meals should avoid excessive fats or tough-to-digest foods, focusing instead on easily digestible ingredients that provide the energy and nutrients necessary for healing.

Proteins like grilled chicken, baked salmon, or tender poached fish are ideal choices, as they are gentle on the stomach and offer essential amino acids that help repair tissues and support immune function. Pairing these proteins with nutrient-rich, easily digestible vegetables such as mashed sweet potatoes, steamed asparagus, or broccoli ensures a well-rounded, nutrient-dense meal. These vegetables provide fiber in forms that are less likely to irritate the gut, especially when they are cooked to a soft consistency. Whole grains like quinoa also make an excellent addition, providing fiber without causing discomfort, and they are a good source of plant-based protein and essential vitamins.

These hearty dinners should focus on light, wholesome ingredients that keep the stomach calm while offering both comfort and nutrition. Meals that combine lean protein, vegetables, and easily digestible grains help promote digestive healing and provide the body with the energy it needs for the long term. These dinners are designed to be satisfying, nourishing, and well-suited for individuals managing digestive conditions while ensuring they can enjoy flavorful and fulfilling meals.

Chicken and Spinach Stew with Soft Carrots

This comforting and nutritious stew is a perfect option for individuals in the recovery phase of diverticulitis. It's gentle on the digestive system, providing lean protein from chicken, fiber from spinach, and vitamins from carrots. The soft vegetables and tender chicken make this dish easy to digest while offering essential nutrients that support healing and overall gut health.

Ingredients:

- 2 chicken breasts, boneless and skinless

- 4 large carrots, peeled and sliced

- 2 cups fresh spinach, washed and chopped

- 1 medium onion, finely chopped

- 2 garlic cloves, minced

- 4 cups low-sodium chicken broth

- 1 tablespoon olive oil

- Salt and pepper to taste

- Fresh herbs like thyme or parsley (optional)

Instructions:

1. Cook the Chicken: In a large pot, heat olive oil over medium heat. Season the chicken breasts with salt and pepper, then cook them in the pot until

browned on both sides. Remove the chicken and set aside to cool.

2. Prepare the Stew Base: In the same pot, add the chopped onion and garlic. Sauté until softened and fragrant, about 3-4 minutes. Add the chicken broth and bring the mixture to a simmer.

3. Cook the Carrots: Add the sliced carrots to the pot and simmer for about 10 minutes until they begin to soften.

4. Shred the Chicken: While the carrots cook, shred the cooked chicken breasts into bite-sized pieces. Once the carrots are tender, add the shredded chicken back into the pot.

5. Add the Spinach: Stir in the chopped spinach and cook for an additional 2-3 minutes until wilted.

6. Season: Taste and adjust the seasoning with additional salt and pepper, if necessary. Optionally, sprinkle with fresh herbs like thyme or parsley.

7. Serve: Ladle the stew into bowls and serve warm.

This Chicken and Spinach Stew with Soft Carrots is an easy-to-digest, nutrient-packed meal that's both soothing and satisfying. It's perfect for those seeking a balanced dinner that supports digestive health while still being rich in flavor and texture.

Baked Salmon with Roasted Root Vegetables

This simple yet flavorful dish combines omega-3 rich salmon with a medley of roasted root vegetables, offering a nutritious, easy-to-digest meal ideal for individuals in the maintenance phase of diverticulitis. The salmon provides high-quality protein and healthy fats that help reduce inflammation, while the soft, roasted root vegetables like carrots, parsnips, and sweet potatoes offer fiber in a gentle form that is less likely to irritate the digestive tract.

Ingredients:

- 2 salmon fillets

- 3 medium carrots, peeled and cut into chunks

- 2 medium sweet potatoes, peeled and cubed

- 1 parsnip, peeled and cut into chunks

- 2 tablespoons olive oil

- 1 teaspoon dried thyme

- Salt and pepper to taste

- 1 tablespoon lemon juice (optional)

- Fresh parsley for garnish (optional)

Instructions:

1. Prepare the Vegetables: Preheat your oven to 400°F (200°C). Place the carrots, sweet potatoes, and parsnip chunks on a baking sheet. Drizzle with

138

olive oil, sprinkle with thyme, salt, and pepper, and toss to coat evenly. Roast for about 25-30 minutes, or until tender, stirring halfway through.

2. Prepare the Salmon: While the vegetables are roasting, season the salmon fillets with salt and pepper. Optionally, drizzle a bit of olive oil or lemon juice on top for extra flavor.

3. Bake the Salmon: After the vegetables have been roasting for about 15-20 minutes, add the salmon fillets to the baking sheet, placing them alongside the vegetables. Bake for an additional 12-15 minutes, or until the salmon is cooked through and flakes easily with a fork.

4. Serve: Once the salmon and vegetables are ready, plate them together and garnish with fresh parsley for a pop of color and added freshness.

This Baked Salmon with Roasted Root Vegetables is not only rich in healthy fats and fiber but also offers a satisfying meal that supports digestive health and provides essential nutrients for long-term well-being. The tender vegetables and perfectly cooked salmon create a balanced, soothing meal that's both nutritious and easy to digest.

Brown Rice and Sautéed Vegetables with Lemon

This simple and nourishing dish combines the wholesome goodness of brown rice with a variety of sautéed vegetables, lightly seasoned with lemon to add a refreshing touch. It's a versatile, fiber-rich meal that's easy on the digestive system, making it an excellent option for those in the recovery or maintenance phase of diverticulitis. Brown rice provides soluble fiber, while the sautéed vegetables offer additional vitamins and antioxidants, making this dish a well-rounded choice to support digestive health.

Ingredients:

- 1 cup brown rice

- 2 tablespoons olive oil

- 1 medium zucchini, sliced

- 1 bell pepper, chopped

- 1 medium carrot, sliced

- 1 cup spinach or kale, chopped

- 1 tablespoon lemon juice

- Salt and pepper to taste

- Fresh parsley or basil for garnish (optional)

Instructions:

1. Cook the Brown Rice: Start by cooking the brown rice according to the package instructions. Typically, brown rice takes about 35-40 minutes to cook. Once done, set it aside.

2. Sauté the Vegetables: In a large skillet, heat the olive oil over medium heat. Add the zucchini, bell pepper, and carrot, and sauté for about 5-7 minutes until tender but still slightly crisp. Add the spinach or

kale and sauté for an additional 1-2 minutes until wilted.

3. Combine the Rice and Vegetables: Once the vegetables are cooked, stir in the cooked brown rice. Drizzle with lemon juice, and season with salt and pepper to taste. Stir well to combine the flavors.

4. Serve: Plate the rice and vegetable mixture, and garnish with fresh herbs like parsley or basil, if desired. Serve warm.

This Brown Rice and Sautéed Vegetables with Lemon is a light, flavorful, and nutrient-packed meal that's gentle on the stomach. It provides fiber for digestive health while also offering essential vitamins and minerals to support long-term well-being. The touch of lemon adds brightness, enhancing the flavors without overwhelming the digestive system.

Healthy Snacks and Desserts

For individuals managing diverticulitis, snacks and desserts can still be enjoyable and nourishing without being harsh on the digestive system. These treats focus on gentle ingredients and natural sweetness while avoiding high-fat, high-sugar, or overly processed items that may trigger discomfort. The following ideas offer a balance of fiber, gentle proteins, and anti-inflammatory ingredients to satisfy cravings while supporting digestive health.

Snack Ideas

1. Greek Yogurt with Softened Fruit: A serving of Greek yogurt with a spoonful of mashed, cooked fruit like apples or pears makes for a creamy and soothing snack. Greek yogurt provides probiotics for gut health, while the fruit adds natural sweetness and fiber in a gentle form.

2. Cottage Cheese with Cucumber and Herbs: Cottage cheese is easy to digest and offers a good source of protein. Add diced cucumber and a

sprinkle of fresh dill or parsley for added flavor without added sugars or irritants.

3. Nut Butter on Rice Cakes: Spread almond or peanut butter on a rice cake for a crunchy, satisfying snack. Nut butters are rich in healthy fats and protein, while rice cakes are easy on the stomach. Choose smooth nut butter without added sugars for a gentle option.

4. Avocado and Banana Mash: Blend half an avocado with a ripe banana for a creamy, nutrient-dense snack. Both avocado and banana offer potassium and healthy fats, while their soft textures make them gentle on the digestive tract.

Dessert Ideas

1. Baked Apples with Cinnamon: Core and slice an apple, sprinkle with cinnamon, and bake until soft. This naturally sweet and fiber-rich dessert is gentle on the digestive system and free of refined sugars.

2. Rice Pudding with Almond Milk: A comforting and simple treat, rice pudding made with almond milk and a dash of vanilla extract is creamy and easy to digest. Lightly sweetened with honey, it provides a gentle dessert option without dairy or excessive sugars.

3. Chia Pudding with Coconut Milk: Chia seeds are an excellent source of omega-3s and fiber. Soak them in coconut milk overnight and enjoy a thick, pudding-like consistency with a touch of honey or maple syrup for sweetness. The coconut milk adds richness, while chia seeds provide a gentle texture.

4. Smoothie Popsicles: Blend a gentle smoothie with ingredients like banana, yogurt, and berries, then pour the mixture into molds and freeze. These popsicles are refreshing and can be customized with ingredients that soothe the digestive system.

5. Banana and Oat Cookies: Mix mashed banana with oats and bake until golden for a naturally sweet treat. These cookies are free of added sugars and are easy on digestion, providing fiber and natural

sugars for energy without the heaviness of traditional baked goods.

These healthy snacks and desserts are designed to be satisfying and gentle, providing options that fit well with a maintenance diet for diverticulitis. They use whole, minimally processed ingredients to provide a balance of flavor, texture, and nutrition, ensuring enjoyment without compromising digestive health.

Steamed Apple Slices with Honey and Cinnamon

This simple yet comforting dessert brings out the natural sweetness of apples while keeping them gentle on the digestive system. Steaming the apples makes them soft and easy to digest, perfect for those managing digestive health. A touch of honey and cinnamon adds warmth and sweetness, turning this dish into a soothing treat that's both delicious and nutritious.

Ingredients:

- 1 large apple (such as Fuji or Honeycrisp), peeled and thinly sliced

- 1 tablespoon honey (optional, to taste)

- 1/4 teaspoon ground cinnamon

- A small pinch of salt (optional)

Instructions:

1. Prepare the Apple Slices: Peel the apple and cut it into thin slices. Peeling and slicing helps make the apples more digestible and speeds up the steaming process.

2. Steam the Apples: Place the apple slices in a steamer basket over a pot of boiling water. Cover and steam for about 5-7 minutes, or until the apples are tender and easily pierced with a fork.

3. Add Honey and Cinnamon: Transfer the steamed apple slices to a bowl. Drizzle with honey and

sprinkle with cinnamon. If desired, add a tiny pinch of salt to enhance the flavors.

4. Serve: Enjoy warm as a gentle dessert or snack.

This dish provides a naturally sweet and fiber-friendly option, perfect for satisfying a sweet craving without overloading the digestive system. The apples are soft and comforting, while cinnamon adds a hint of spice that complements their sweetness.

Chia Pudding with Almond Milk

Chia pudding is a versatile, nutritious treat that's gentle on the digestive system and packed with fiber, omega-3s, and protein. Made with almond milk and naturally sweetened, it's a great option for anyone looking for a soothing snack or dessert that also supports gut health.

Ingredients:

- 3 tablespoons chia seeds

- 1 cup unsweetened almond milk

- 1-2 teaspoons honey or maple syrup (optional, to taste)

- 1/4 teaspoon vanilla extract (optional)

Instructions:

1. Combine Ingredients: In a bowl or jar, mix the chia seeds, almond milk, sweetener, and vanilla extract, if using. Stir well to ensure the chia seeds are fully immersed in the liquid.

2. Let It Sit: Cover the bowl or jar and refrigerate for at least 2 hours, or ideally overnight. This allows the chia seeds to absorb the almond milk and thicken into a pudding-like consistency.

3. Stir and Serve: Once the pudding has set, give it a good stir to break up any clumps. Serve chilled, topped with soft fruits like mashed banana or stewed berries, if desired.

This chia pudding is light, creamy, and satisfying, providing a gentle way to enjoy fiber and healthy fats. The almond milk and honey create a mildly sweet base, while chia seeds add a unique texture, making it a balanced snack or dessert option for digestive health.

Soft Baked Sweet Potato Chips with Olive Oil

These soft, baked sweet potato chips are a nutritious and gentle snack option, perfect for individuals needing easy-to-digest foods. Unlike traditional crunchy chips, these baked sweet potato slices are tender, making them suitable for those managing digestive health while still providing fiber, vitamins, and a bit of healthy fat.

Ingredients:

- 1 large sweet potato, peeled and thinly sliced (about 1/8-inch thick)

- 1-2 tablespoons olive oil

- A pinch of sea salt (optional)

- A sprinkle of cinnamon or rosemary (optional, for added flavor)

Instructions:

1. Prepare the Sweet Potato: Preheat your oven to 350°F (175°C). Line a baking sheet with parchment paper. Peel and slice the sweet potato into thin, even slices. A mandoline slicer can help achieve uniform thickness, but a knife works well, too.

2. Season and Oil: In a large bowl, toss the sweet potato slices with olive oil, ensuring each slice is lightly coated. Sprinkle with a pinch of salt and any other desired seasonings, such as cinnamon for sweetness or rosemary for a savory twist.

3. Bake: Arrange the sweet potato slices in a single layer on the baking sheet. Bake for 20-25 minutes, flipping halfway through, until the slices are soft and tender. Keep an eye on them to avoid over-browning.

4. Serve: Let the chips cool slightly before serving. They're best enjoyed warm, either as a snack or a side dish.

These soft baked sweet potato chips are delicious and nourishing, offering a gentle texture and natural sweetness. The olive oil adds a light crispiness and healthy fats, making this snack both enjoyable and easy on the stomach.

Chapter 5

Meal Plans for Digestive Health

Meal planning is a key aspect of supporting digestive health, especially for those dealing with conditions like diverticulitis. A carefully crafted meal plan ensures you get the essential nutrients you need without overloading the digestive system. In this chapter, we'll explore tailored meal plans that support different phases of digestive wellness, including flare-up, recovery, and long-term maintenance. Each plan is designed with a focus on balance, ease of digestion, and anti-inflammatory ingredients, making it easier to follow dietary recommendations and reduce digestive strain.

During the flare-up phase, the goal is to minimize digestive irritation by choosing soothing, low-residue foods. Clear broths, gentle soups, and pureed foods are emphasized, giving the digestive system a break and promoting healing. These foods are nutritious yet light, offering the body much-needed energy without triggering discomfort.

As symptoms begin to improve, the recovery phase introduces soft, low-fiber foods that gently support healing without overwhelming the digestive system. Cooked vegetables, peeled fruits, and lean proteins are highlighted, ensuring a balance of vitamins and nutrients while still being easy to digest. This phase is all about gradually reintroducing foods in a way that encourages the digestive system to strengthen and return to regular function.

For long-term maintenance, high-fiber and anti-inflammatory foods become central. This phase emphasizes the inclusion of whole grains, lean proteins, and a variety of fruits and vegetables to support gut health and reduce the risk of future flare-ups. By incorporating fiber, antioxidants, and anti-inflammatory nutrients, this plan promotes ongoing digestive wellness, helping to build a strong foundation for overall health.

Each meal plan is designed to meet the changing needs of the digestive system, offering a supportive and structured approach to eating for improved gut health. Whether you're managing a flare-up, recovering, or focusing on long-term health, these meal plans provide the flexibility and variety needed to nourish the body while respecting digestive sensitivities.

Flare-Up Phase: 3-Day Liquid and Low-Residue Plan

During a diverticulitis flare-up, a liquid and low-residue diet can help ease symptoms and give your digestive system a chance to rest. This gentle approach focuses on clear liquids, nutrient-rich broths, and easily digestible foods, providing hydration, essential nutrients, and comfort without irritating the inflamed areas. Below is a suggested 3-day meal plan that includes nourishing options designed to support you through this phase.

Day 1: Liquid Phase

Breakfast: Clear apple juice and herbal tea (such as chamomile or peppermint)
Mid-Morning: Warm vegetable broth with parsley
Lunch: Strained carrot and ginger soup

Afternoon Snack: Coconut water or electrolyte-infused water
Dinner: Bone broth with a hint of ginger for added flavor and soothing properties
Evening: Chamomile tea

This first day focuses on clear liquids to reduce any digestive strain. Vegetable broth, herbal teas, and bone broth provide warmth, comfort, and essential minerals to keep your body nourished as you ease through symptoms.

Day 2: Transitioning to Low-Residue Liquids

Breakfast: Electrolyte-infused water with cucumber and mint, plus strained apple and ginger juice
Mid-Morning: Clear cucumber and melon juice
Lunch: Strained vegetable broth, adding in a bit of potato for more substance if well-tolerated
Afternoon Snack: Hydrating coconut water smoothie (strained)
Dinner: Gentle carrot and potato broth, carefully strained
Evening: Peppermint tea to aid digestion

The second day allows for gentle, nutrient-dense broths and low-fiber liquids, building a little more sustenance as symptoms allow. This helps prepare the digestive system to start reintroducing soft foods.

Day 3: Introducing Pureed and Soft Low-Residue Foods

Breakfast: Smooth rice porridge with coconut milk
Mid-Morning: Clear chamomile tea or mild peppermint tea
Lunch: Pureed potato and leek soup, well-strained and thin in consistency
Afternoon Snack: Coconut water or a clear, hydrating juice option
Dinner: Strained carrot and ginger soup with bone broth base
Evening: Warm chamomile tea

By Day 3, you're gradually moving to thicker liquids, incorporating lightly pureed options that remain low in fiber yet provide additional nourishment. This gentle approach continues to support hydration and healing, with the addition of soft foods helping prepare your body for more variety as you begin to recover.

This 3-day flare-up plan prioritizes hydration, essential nutrients, and rest for your digestive system, offering a foundation of gentle foods to soothe and support recovery. As you start to feel better, you can slowly transition into the recovery phase with soft, low-fiber foods in small portions, gradually expanding your diet based on your tolerance and comfort level.

Recovery Phase: 5-Day Soft Foods Plan

After a flare-up, transitioning to soft, low-fiber foods can help ease your digestive system back into regular functioning without overwhelming it. The goal in this phase is to reintroduce nourishing foods that are easy to digest, low in fiber, and gentle on the stomach, while still providing the nutrients your body needs to support healing and recovery.

Day 1: Gentle Start with Soft Foods

Breakfast: Creamy oatmeal made with water or almond milk, topped with a small amount of strained applesauce
Mid-Morning: Warm chamomile tea

Lunch: Smooth potato and leek puree

Afternoon Snack: Applesauce with a hint of cinnamon

Dinner: Pureed carrot and zucchini soup with a bit of olive oil for extra flavor and nutrition

Evening: Peppermint tea to soothe digestion

Day 2: Introducing Mild Proteins

Breakfast: Soft-boiled egg with a small side of steamed spinach (chopped for easy digestion)

Mid-Morning: Mild herbal tea (such as ginger or chamomile)

Lunch: Soft mashed sweet potatoes with a dash of olive oil

Afternoon Snack: Banana and pear puree, ensuring a smooth consistency

Dinner: Poached chicken breast with pureed carrots and a touch of herbs like parsley

Evening: Peppermint tea

Day 3: Expanding Flavors and Textures

Breakfast: Smooth rice porridge made with coconut milk

Mid-Morning: Warm tea or electrolyte-infused water

Lunch: Scrambled eggs with a small amount of finely chopped fresh herbs like dill or parsley
Afternoon Snack: Soft mashed avocado with a little lemon juice, eaten plain or spread on a rice cake if well-tolerated
Dinner: Steamed and mashed cauliflower with a bit of garlic, alongside soft-baked white fish (such as cod)
Evening: Chamomile tea

Day 4: Adding a Bit More Fiber and Variety

Breakfast: Overnight oats (cooked well and softened) with a small portion of steamed berries (such as blueberries)
Mid-Morning: Peppermint tea or chamomile tea
Lunch: Mashed lentils with pureed pumpkin, seasoned lightly with turmeric
Afternoon Snack: Applesauce mixed with a little bit of honey (if desired)
Dinner: Baked salmon with mashed butternut squash and steamed green beans (mashed if needed for easier digestion)
Evening: Ginger tea

Day 5: Preparing for a Balanced Diet

Breakfast: Greek yogurt with a softened, diced pear (or pureed if preferred) and a drizzle of honey
Mid-Morning: Coconut water for hydration
Lunch: Soft quinoa with cooked, mashed vegetables like carrots and zucchini, drizzled with olive oil
Afternoon Snack: Chia pudding made with almond milk, kept at a soft, smooth consistency
Dinner: Stewed chicken with pureed sweet potatoes and steamed spinach (chopped for easy digestion)
Evening: Chamomile tea to end the day

In this 5-day soft foods plan, the focus is on gentle, low-fiber foods that help your digestive system recover without strain. Each day gradually increases variety and nutrition, allowing your digestive system to adjust to new foods and textures at a steady, comfortable pace. Once you're feeling stronger and your body is ready, you can start reintroducing more fiber-rich foods slowly, building up to a well-balanced diet that supports long-term gut health.

Maintenance Phase: 7-Day High-Fiber, Anti-Inflammatory Plan

The maintenance phase focuses on incorporating high-fiber and anti-inflammatory foods to promote long-term digestive health and prevent future flare-ups. High-fiber foods aid in regular digestion and add bulk to the stool, helping to prevent the development of new diverticula. Anti-inflammatory foods can reduce inflammation, promoting overall gut health. This 7-day plan balances fiber with easy-to-digest nutrients, gradually enhancing gut resilience.

Day 1: Simple Start to Fiber-Rich Eating

Breakfast: Overnight oats with chia seeds and a small amount of honey
Lunch: Quinoa and mixed greens with shredded carrots, diced cucumber, and olive oil dressing
Dinner: Baked salmon with mashed sweet potatoes and steamed green beans
Snack Options: Softened pear or banana, raw almonds (if tolerated)

Day 2: Adding Anti-Inflammatory Ingredients

Breakfast: Greek yogurt with ground flaxseed and softened berries

Lunch: Lentil soup with carrots, celery, and a sprinkle of turmeric
Dinner: Brown rice with sautéed spinach and baked chicken breast, seasoned with rosemary
Snack Options: Hummus with soft veggies like steamed baby carrots or bell peppers

Day 3: Gradually Increasing Fiber

Breakfast: Smoothie with spinach, banana, chia seeds, and a small amount of almond milk
Lunch: Mixed grain bowl with farro, roasted vegetables, and a sprinkle of pumpkin seeds
Dinner: Stir-fried tofu with broccoli, bell peppers, and a light ginger-garlic sauce
Snack Options: Apple slices with almond butter

Day 4: Emphasizing Anti-Inflammatory Herbs and Spices

Breakfast: Oatmeal with a pinch of cinnamon, chopped apple, and a spoonful of flaxseed
Lunch: Chickpea and vegetable stew with diced tomatoes, zucchini, and turmeric
Dinner: Grilled cod with a side of roasted Brussels sprouts and mashed cauliflower

Snack Options: Handful of walnuts or a cucumber-mint infused water

Day 5: Variety and Flavor with High-Fiber Options

Breakfast: Chia pudding made with almond milk and topped with a few blueberries
Lunch: Soft black bean and sweet potato salad with lime and cilantro dressing
Dinner: Spaghetti squash with tomato-basil sauce and a side of steamed spinach
Snack Options: Softened apricots or dates (in moderation)

Day 6: Adding Nutrient-Dense Greens

Breakfast: Smoothie bowl with mixed greens, banana, ground chia, and almond milk
Lunch: Barley and roasted vegetable salad with olive oil and a sprinkle of sesame seeds
Dinner: Baked chicken with mashed carrots and sautéed kale
Snack Options: Baby carrots with tahini dressing

Day 7: Balanced High-Fiber and Anti-Inflammatory Meals

Breakfast: Oatmeal with raspberries, ground flaxseed, and a touch of honey
Lunch: Wild rice with diced bell peppers, chopped spinach, and chickpeas, drizzled with a light vinaigrette
Dinner: Lentil-stuffed bell pepper with a side of steamed asparagus
Snack Options: Sliced cucumber or avocado with a dash of sea salt

This 7-day plan provides balanced, high-fiber, and anti-inflammatory meals that support digestive health. It focuses on fresh, minimally processed foods to nourish your body and keep your gut in good condition. Always adjust portions and specific ingredients to your tolerance and consult with a healthcare provider to tailor this plan further if needed.

Tips on adjusting the meal plans based on individual tolerance

Adjusting meal plans based on individual tolerance is key to managing diverticulitis and maintaining digestive health. While the 7-day high-fiber, anti-inflammatory plan provides a solid foundation, it's essential to tailor it to your body's specific needs and reactions. Here are some tips to help you make adjustments based on your tolerance:

1. Gradual Introduction of Fiber:

If you're sensitive to fiber, introduce it gradually to avoid overwhelming your digestive system. Start with smaller portions of high-fiber foods, like oatmeal, quinoa, and vegetables, and increase the portion sizes as your body becomes accustomed to them.

Tip: If you experience discomfort after eating high-fiber foods, reduce the amount and reintroduce them more slowly. You can also try soaking or cooking grains and beans to make them gentler on your digestive system.

2. Monitor Sensitivity to Raw Vegetables:

Raw vegetables, especially cruciferous ones like broccoli and cauliflower, can be hard to digest for some people with diverticulitis. If this is the case, opt for steamed or cooked versions of these vegetables instead.

Tip: Use cooking methods like steaming, roasting, or sautéing to soften vegetables and make them easier to digest. You can also peel and deseed vegetables like tomatoes and cucumbers to reduce their fiber content.

3. Choose Low-FODMAP Alternatives:

Some people with digestive conditions like diverticulitis may be sensitive to high-FODMAP foods (fermentable oligosaccharides, disaccharides, monosaccharides, and polyols), which can cause bloating and discomfort.

Tip: If you experience bloating or gas, try eliminating common high-FODMAP foods like garlic, onions, and certain fruits. Substitute them with low-FODMAP options such as zucchini, carrots, and spinach.

4. Adjust Protein Sources:

Lean proteins like chicken, fish, and tofu are generally easier to digest, but if you have trouble digesting meat or find it heavy on your stomach, consider plant-based proteins like lentils or beans in smaller amounts.

Tip: If legumes cause bloating, try soaking and cooking them well or using canned versions with a rinse to reduce gas-producing compounds.

5. Avoid Trigger Foods:

Every individual has different food triggers. Common irritants for people with diverticulitis include spicy foods, fatty foods, and processed items.

Tip: Keep track of any foods that cause flare-ups and adjust the meal plan to exclude them. Focus on whole, unprocessed foods for the best results.

6. Hydrate Well:

Fiber requires adequate hydration to aid digestion. If you increase fiber, be sure to drink plenty of water throughout the day to avoid constipation.

Tip: Include hydrating beverages like herbal teas or infused water to keep your body hydrated, and adjust your fluid intake based on your activity level and fiber consumption.

7. Portion Control:

Large meals may put a strain on your digestive system. It's often better to eat smaller, more frequent meals throughout the day.

Tip: Pay attention to portion sizes and avoid overeating, especially when reintroducing new foods or ingredients. Eating slowly and mindfully can also help reduce digestive discomfort.

8. Experiment with Fermented Foods:

Some individuals find that fermented foods like yogurt or kefir help balance gut bacteria and improve digestion. However, others may find them too rich or acidic.

Tip: Start with small amounts of fermented foods and assess your tolerance. If you feel discomfort, reduce the amount or try alternatives like non-dairy probiotics.

By paying attention to your body's signals and gradually making these adjustments, you can customize the meal plan to fit your unique digestive needs, while still prioritizing fiber, anti-inflammatory foods, and overall gut health.

Chapter 6

Navigating Everyday Challenges with Diverticulitis

Living with diverticulitis can bring its set of daily challenges, especially when trying to maintain a balanced diet while managing flare-ups. This chapter focuses on practical strategies for navigating everyday situations that may arise while living with diverticulitis, from dining out and grocery shopping to managing stress and maintaining a social life. By providing tips, tricks, and real-life solutions, this chapter will empower you to take control of your health and minimize the impact of diverticulitis on your daily life.

Dealing with Flare-Ups While Out and About Managing diverticulitis flare-ups often requires careful planning, especially when you're out in public. Whether you're at work, traveling, or attending social gatherings, it's important to know how to manage flare-ups and still enjoy life. This section will offer advice on handling flare-ups in public settings, including identifying safe food choices when dining out, and how to politely decline foods that might irritate your digestive system. You'll also learn how to cope with flare-ups while away from home, including tips for meal prepping and keeping a stash of easy-to-digest snacks in your bag or car.

Grocery Shopping with Diverticulitis
When living with diverticulitis, grocery shopping requires extra thought and preparation. This section will provide a comprehensive guide on what to look for when shopping for foods that support digestive health. From fiber-friendly options to anti-inflammatory ingredients, you'll get a breakdown of key food items to keep in your pantry and refrigerator. You'll also learn how to read labels and avoid hidden additives or preservatives that could potentially cause discomfort.

Maintaining Social Connections
Social gatherings and meals with friends and family can be a source of stress for people with diverticulitis, particularly when food choices may be limited. This section will offer helpful tips for navigating social events and gatherings without feeling excluded or anxious. Whether it's attending a dinner party or enjoying a meal at a friend's

house, you'll learn how to communicate your dietary needs with loved ones and make adjustments to enjoy the social aspect of the occasion without sacrificing your health.

Managing Stress and Emotional Well-being
Stress can be a major trigger for diverticulitis flare-ups. This section will provide strategies for managing stress in everyday life, such as practicing mindfulness, yoga, or other relaxation techniques. Maintaining a calm and centered mindset can reduce flare-ups and contribute to better overall digestive health. Additionally, we'll address the importance of getting adequate sleep, staying hydrated, and listening to your body's signals.

By using the tips and strategies outlined in this chapter, you'll be better equipped to navigate the everyday challenges of living with diverticulitis while still enjoying a fulfilling, balanced life.

Dining Out with Confidence

Dining out with diverticulitis can sometimes feel like navigating a minefield. With the wrong food choices, a meal at a restaurant can trigger a flare-up, leaving you feeling uncomfortable or even in pain. However, with a bit of planning and confidence, you can enjoy social meals without compromising your health. This section will offer practical tips and strategies to help you dine out with confidence while managing your condition.

Research Before You Go

One of the easiest ways to ensure a positive dining experience is to research the restaurant beforehand. Many restaurants now offer menus online, and some even highlight specific dietary options. Look for establishments that offer meals suited for your dietary needs, such as gluten-free, low-residue, or anti-inflammatory options. Some restaurants might even allow you to call ahead to discuss your dietary restrictions or make adjustments to your order.

Know What to Avoid

When dining out, it's important to be aware of the foods that can trigger flare-ups. Typically, high-fiber foods, such as seeds, nuts, and raw vegetables, should be avoided, as well as fatty or fried foods, which can irritate the digestive system. Foods that are spicy or overly seasoned might also cause discomfort. Steer clear of dishes that contain heavy cream or rich sauces, as these can be too hard to digest during a flare-up.

Simple and Customizable Choices

Opt for simple, easily customizable dishes like grilled chicken, steamed vegetables, or soups without added dairy or cream. Many restaurants are accommodating and can make small changes to dishes, such as removing or substituting ingredients to suit your needs. For example, you could request that your vegetables be steamed instead of sautéed or ask for dressing on the side to control the amount used. If you're unsure about something on the menu, don't hesitate to ask your server for clarification or alternative suggestions.

Bring Your Own Snacks

If you're heading out to a social gathering or a restaurant where options are limited, consider bringing your own safe, easy-to-digest snacks. Simple choices like pre-packaged applesauce, homemade smoothies, or plain crackers can ensure that you won't go hungry if the restaurant's offerings don't suit your needs. Having snacks on hand can help you feel more confident and prepared.

Practice Mindful Eating

When dining out, it's important to practice mindful eating—eat slowly, savor each bite, and listen to your body. This approach will allow you to tune into your digestive system, making it easier to identify any discomfort or warning signs that might indicate a flare-up. Eating slowly can also improve digestion and reduce the risk of overeating or consuming too much food that may aggravate your condition.

Communication is Key

It's essential to communicate your dietary restrictions to your server. Most restaurants are willing to accommodate special dietary needs, and by being clear about what you can or cannot eat, you can ensure that your meal is prepared in a way that supports your health. It might feel awkward at first, but advocating for yourself will ultimately help you enjoy your dining experience with fewer worries.

Enjoy the Experience

Dining out isn't just about the food—it's about the experience and connection with others. With these tips, you can still enjoy socializing with friends and family while being mindful of your dietary restrictions. Embrace the opportunity to try new foods that align with your digestive needs and take pleasure in the social aspect of dining out.

By being proactive, staying informed, and making mindful choices, you can confidently navigate dining out with diverticulitis, ensuring that every meal is both enjoyable and supportive of your digestive health.

Safely Reintroducing Foods

Reintroducing foods after a diverticulitis flare-up requires patience, attention, and careful planning. The digestive system can be sensitive during this phase, and the wrong foods can cause discomfort or even lead to another flare-up. Gradually reintroducing foods ensures that your body can handle the changes without overloading the digestive system. Here are some important steps and considerations for safely reintroducing foods to your diet.

Start Slow and Steady
After a flare-up, your digestive system may be more sensitive. It's important to introduce foods slowly,

starting with simple, easy-to-digest options. Begin with foods that are soft and low in fiber, such as well-cooked vegetables, mashed potatoes, and lean proteins like chicken or fish. These foods are gentle on the stomach and can help your digestive system ease back into regular function.

Introduce One Food at a Time
To monitor your body's reaction, introduce one food at a time and wait a couple of days before adding another. This allows you to track how each food affects your digestive system. If a particular food causes discomfort, bloating, or gas, it may not yet be suitable for reintroduction. It's essential to listen to your body's signals and avoid rushing the process.

Gradually Increase Fiber
Fiber plays a key role in digestive health, but after a flare-up, it's crucial to gradually increase fiber intake to avoid overwhelming the system. Start with soft, well-cooked, or pureed vegetables and fruits. As your body adjusts, you can slowly introduce higher-fiber foods, such as cooked whole grains, oatmeal, and legumes. Avoid raw fruits and vegetables, as they can be harder to digest and may cause irritation.

Be Cautious with Seeds and Nuts
For individuals with diverticulitis, seeds and nuts can sometimes trigger flare-ups, especially during the early stages of recovery. While some research suggests that consuming seeds and nuts in moderation may be safe for many, it's still wise to avoid them initially. If you'd like to reintroduce them, begin with small amounts and observe how your body responds.

Avoid Trigger Foods
Some foods are more likely to trigger flare-ups and should be avoided during the reintroduction phase. These include spicy foods, caffeine, alcohol, and foods high in fat, which can be irritating to the digestive tract. Similarly, avoid foods that are overly processed or contain additives and preservatives, as they can aggravate symptoms. Stick to whole, minimally processed foods that are easy on the gut.

Hydration is Key
During the reintroduction phase, staying hydrated is essential to support the digestive process and help your body adjust. Water, herbal teas, and clear broths are excellent options to keep you hydrated. Coconut water can also help replenish electrolytes.

It's important to drink plenty of fluids to aid digestion and prevent constipation as you begin reintroducing solid foods.

Monitor Your Body's Response
Keep a food journal during this process to track your meals, symptoms, and any reactions you experience. This can help you identify any problematic foods and give you a better understanding of which foods support your digestive health. If you notice any adverse symptoms, like bloating, pain, or discomfort, consult with a healthcare professional before reintroducing those foods.

Seek Professional Guidance
If you're unsure about how to safely reintroduce foods, it's always a good idea to consult with a dietitian or healthcare provider. They can offer personalized guidance based on your specific needs and health condition. They may also recommend specific foods or supplements to support gut health as you transition back to a regular diet.

By carefully reintroducing foods and monitoring how your body responds, you can safely recover from a diverticulitis flare-up and return to a balanced, healthy diet. The key is to proceed slowly, stay mindful of your body's signals, and avoid foods that may cause irritation or discomfort. With time and attention, you'll be able to expand your food choices and enjoy a varied and nourishing diet once again.

Special Dietary Considerations

When managing diverticulitis, there are certain dietary considerations that may need to be addressed based on individual health needs, lifestyle, or additional conditions. Special dietary needs can vary greatly from person to person, so it's important to be mindful of any other health conditions you may have, along with how your digestive system reacts to different foods. Below are some key special dietary considerations for individuals with diverticulitis:

Low FODMAP Diet
The Low FODMAP diet, which stands for fermentable oligosaccharides, disaccharides, monosaccharides, and polyols, is often recommended for individuals with digestive issues

like IBS (irritable bowel syndrome) or diverticulitis. These types of carbohydrates can be poorly absorbed in the small intestine, causing bloating, gas, and abdominal pain. Many people with diverticulitis benefit from reducing high-FODMAP foods such as onions, garlic, wheat, certain fruits (like apples and cherries), and dairy. Working with a dietitian can help tailor this diet to your needs and ensure you're still getting enough nutrients.

Food Sensitivities and Allergies
Some individuals with diverticulitis may have food sensitivities or allergies that can further irritate the digestive system. Common culprits include dairy, gluten, or certain artificial additives and preservatives. If you suspect a food sensitivity, it's helpful to eliminate these foods from your diet temporarily and monitor any improvements in your symptoms. Reintroduce foods one by one to identify triggers and work with a healthcare provider to confirm any allergies.

Anti-Inflammatory Diet
An anti-inflammatory diet is particularly important for people managing chronic conditions like diverticulitis. Certain foods can promote inflammation, while others have anti-inflammatory

properties that may help with healing and reducing flare-ups. Foods rich in omega-3 fatty acids, such as salmon, flaxseeds, and walnuts, along with antioxidant-rich fruits and vegetables (e.g., berries, spinach, and kale), can help reduce inflammation in the gut. A balanced anti-inflammatory diet can be beneficial for long-term digestive health.

Fiber Intake

As previously mentioned, fiber plays a crucial role in digestive health, but the type of fiber you consume is important. During a flare-up, it's generally recommended to follow a low-residue or low-fiber diet to avoid aggravating the intestines. However, during recovery and the maintenance phase, increasing fiber intake is key. It's important to gradually add fiber back into your diet to avoid discomfort and improve digestion. Focus on soluble fiber, which is gentler on the gut. Sources include oats, carrots, and bananas. Insoluble fiber found in whole grains, raw vegetables, and nuts should be slowly reintroduced based on tolerance.

Hydration

Proper hydration is critical when managing diverticulitis, as dehydration can worsen constipation and exacerbate symptoms. In addition to drinking plenty of water, it's important to stay hydrated with broths, herbal teas, and electrolyte-infused beverages. Staying hydrated helps soften stool, ease digestion, and prevent further flare-ups. Coconut water and homemade electrolyte drinks (with natural ingredients like lemon and cucumber) are excellent choices for replenishing fluids.

Small, Frequent Meals

For individuals with diverticulitis, large meals can put extra pressure on the digestive system and potentially trigger flare-ups. Instead, consider eating smaller, more frequent meals throughout the day to reduce stress on the intestines. This approach can help improve digestion, avoid bloating, and maintain stable blood sugar levels, which is particularly important if you are dealing with any comorbid conditions such as diabetes or high blood pressure.

Vegan or Vegetarian Diets

Some people with diverticulitis may find that a plant-based diet works best for them, as long as it is well-balanced. A vegan or vegetarian diet can offer many health benefits, including high amounts of fiber, antioxidants, and other nutrients. However, it's crucial to ensure you're getting adequate protein and other essential nutrients (like vitamin B12, iron, and calcium) from plant-based sources such as legumes, tofu, lentils, and leafy greens. Careful planning and supplementation may be necessary to avoid nutritional deficiencies.

Consultation with a Dietitian
Since dietary needs vary significantly, especially in individuals with multiple health conditions or complex digestive issues, consulting with a registered dietitian is highly recommended. A dietitian can help you create a tailored meal plan that meets your specific needs, provides essential nutrients, and avoids foods that may trigger diverticulitis flare-ups. They can also offer guidance on balancing fiber intake, managing food sensitivities, and ensuring overall digestive health.

By taking into account these special dietary considerations, you can manage your diverticulitis symptoms more effectively, reduce the likelihood of flare-ups, and promote long-term digestive health. With careful planning and professional guidance, a customized diet can make a significant difference in how you feel day to day and in managing your condition for the future.

Chapter 7

Tools for Long-Term Health

Living with diverticulitis involves more than just managing flare-ups; it requires long-term strategies to maintain overall health and digestive function. A holistic approach is crucial for reducing flare-ups, improving digestive health, and ensuring long-term well-being.

Regular physical activity is essential for promoting digestive health. Gentle exercises like walking, swimming, or yoga can stimulate the digestive system, helping to alleviate constipation and improve gut motility. However, during flare-ups, it is important to choose activities that do not put excessive strain on the abdomen. Exercise should be adjusted to your tolerance levels to support both physical and digestive well-being.

Mindful eating is another valuable practice for maintaining digestive health. Taking time to chew food properly and eating in a calm, relaxed environment can promote better digestion, reduce indigestion, and prevent overconsumption, which can put stress on the digestive system. Slowing down during meals helps you to recognize when you're full, preventing overeating and supporting optimal digestion.

Stress management is vital, as stress can exacerbate digestive issues and trigger flare-ups. Incorporating relaxation techniques such as meditation, deep breathing, and mindfulness can help reduce stress, allowing your digestive system to function more effectively. Chronic stress negatively affects the gut, increasing inflammation and disrupting the microbiome, so addressing it is essential for long-term health.

Maintaining a healthy gut microbiome is also crucial. Probiotics, whether in food or supplements, help support the balance of good bacteria in the gut, reducing inflammation and improving overall digestive health. Fermented foods like yogurt and kefir are excellent sources of probiotics, but it's important to consult with a healthcare provider before beginning supplementation.

Staying hydrated is another fundamental tool. Proper hydration helps keep digestion smooth, prevents constipation, and promotes healthy bowel movements. Drinking plenty of water, herbal teas, and other hydrating beverages ensures that the digestive system functions optimally.

Regular check-ups with healthcare providers are necessary for monitoring your condition and addressing any emerging health concerns. A doctor or gastroenterologist can help manage flare-ups, prevent complications, and adjust treatment plans as needed. Additionally, working with a dietitian can provide guidance in creating a balanced, individualized diet that supports digestive health.

Keeping track of symptoms and food intake through a food journal can help identify triggers and patterns that affect digestive health. Recording these details can help refine diet choices and avoid foods that may cause flare-ups. A symptom diary can also be useful when communicating with healthcare providers to make informed decisions about treatment.

Adequate sleep is essential for healing and maintaining long-term digestive health. Poor sleep can disrupt the gut microbiome and lead to more frequent flare-ups. Prioritizing restful sleep by creating a sleep routine and a calm sleep environment can help restore balance to the body and support digestive health.

In some cases, nutritional supplements such as fiber or omega-3 fatty acids may be beneficial in supporting digestive health. However, supplements should be used under the guidance of a healthcare professional to ensure they are appropriate for individual needs.

Lastly, educating yourself about diverticulitis, dietary strategies, and treatment options empowers you to make informed decisions about your health. Understanding the condition and staying updated on new research will help you manage symptoms, prevent complications, and maintain long-term health.

By incorporating these strategies—exercise, mindful eating, stress management, hydration, regular check-ups, and more—you can effectively manage diverticulitis and support your digestive health for the long term. A holistic approach to health, combining lifestyle changes with professional support, will provide the best opportunity for sustained wellness.

Stress Management Techniques

Managing stress is crucial for individuals with diverticulitis, as stress can exacerbate symptoms, trigger flare-ups, and impact overall digestive health. Effective stress management techniques help maintain balance and support both physical and mental well-being. In this chapter, we'll explore several methods to manage stress, including breathing exercises, meditation, and mindfulness practices, all of which promote relaxation and reduce anxiety.

Breathing Exercises

Deep breathing exercises are one of the most effective ways to manage stress and calm the nervous system. When you're stressed, your body enters a "fight or flight" state, which can lead to tension, digestive upset, and discomfort. Slow, deep breaths activate the parasympathetic nervous system, which promotes relaxation and helps reduce inflammation, a key factor in diverticulitis flare-ups. Here are some simple breathing techniques to try:

1. Diaphragmatic Breathing: Sit or lie down in a comfortable position. Place one hand on your chest and the other on your abdomen. Take a deep breath in through your nose, allowing your abdomen to rise as you fill your lungs with air. Slowly exhale through your mouth, letting your abdomen fall. Repeat this process for several minutes, focusing on slow, steady breaths.

2. 4-7-8 Breathing Technique: Breathe in through your nose for a count of four, hold your breath for a count of seven, and exhale slowly through your mouth for a count of eight. This technique calms the mind and helps lower stress levels.

Meditation

Meditation is a powerful tool for reducing stress and enhancing emotional well-being. By practicing meditation regularly, you can develop greater awareness of your thoughts and emotions, which allows you to respond to stressors with more calm and control. Meditation also promotes relaxation, lowers heart rate, and reduces inflammation in the body.

To start, find a quiet space where you won't be disturbed. Sit comfortably with your back straight and close your eyes. Focus on your breath or choose a mantra or affirmation to repeat. Allow your thoughts to come and go without judgment, gently bringing your focus back to your breath if your mind wanders. Aim to meditate for 5-10 minutes daily, gradually increasing the time as you become more comfortable.

Mindfulness Practices

Mindfulness involves staying present and fully engaged in the current moment, without judgment. This practice can help reduce stress by preventing you from overthinking or worrying about the past or future. Mindfulness encourages you to acknowledge your thoughts, emotions, and physical sensations without becoming overwhelmed by them.

Here are a few simple mindfulness techniques to incorporate into your daily routine:

1. Body Scan Meditation: Lie down in a comfortable position and focus on each part of your body, starting from your toes and moving upward to your head. As you focus on each area, observe any tension or discomfort, and consciously relax that part of your body.

2. Mindful Eating: When eating, pay full attention to the experience. Notice the colors, textures, and flavors of the food. Chew slowly and savor each bite. Mindful eating helps improve digestion, prevent overeating, and cultivate a deeper connection with your body's needs.

3. Grounding Exercises: When you're feeling overwhelmed or stressed, grounding techniques can help you reconnect with the present moment. One simple exercise is to take a deep breath and focus on the physical sensations of your body in contact with the ground or a chair. Notice how your feet feel against the floor or how your body feels supported by the chair.

The Benefits of Stress Management for Diverticulitis

Consistently practicing stress management techniques can help mitigate the impact of stress on your digestive system. Chronic stress can lead to increased inflammation in the gut, disrupting the balance of gut bacteria, impairing digestion, and making diverticulitis flare-ups more likely. By engaging in regular relaxation techniques like breathing exercises, meditation, and mindfulness practices, you can reduce the physical and emotional strain that stress places on your body, promoting healing and overall well-being.

Incorporating these techniques into your daily life can provide a sense of calm and control, enabling you to better manage the challenges of living with diverticulitis. Remember, stress is an inevitable part of life, but how you manage it can make a significant difference in your physical health and emotional resilience.

Tracking Your Symptoms and Progress

Tracking your symptoms and progress is essential for effectively managing diverticulitis. By keeping a detailed record of your symptoms, diet, and lifestyle factors, you can better understand what triggers flare-ups and which strategies help you maintain digestive health. This process also allows you to communicate more effectively with your healthcare team, providing them with valuable insights to adjust your treatment plan if necessary.

To track your symptoms, note when flare-ups occur, their severity, and any accompanying symptoms such as pain, bloating, nausea, or changes in bowel habits. Recording what you eat can help identify potential dietary triggers, such as high-fiber foods or certain spices that may worsen your condition. Additionally, documenting stress levels, sleep quality, and physical activity can provide a clearer picture of how these factors affect your health.

Consider using a journal or an app designed for health tracking to make it easier to monitor your progress over time. This allows you to review patterns, assess how changes in diet or lifestyle impact your symptoms, and make adjustments accordingly. Over time, you'll develop a better understanding of what works best for your body, helping you take proactive steps to prevent flare-ups and manage your condition effectively.

Tips for identifying food triggers and managing symptoms

Identifying food triggers and managing symptoms of diverticulitis involves a combination of observation, trial and error, and making mindful choices about what you eat. Here are some practical tips for recognizing food triggers and managing flare-ups effectively:

Start by keeping a food diary. Write down everything you eat, including the times you eat, and note any symptoms that occur afterward. This will help you identify patterns and potential triggers. Pay close attention to foods that tend to cause discomfort, such as high-fiber items (like nuts, seeds, and whole grains), spicy foods, or fried and fatty meals. Keeping track of your bowel movements, bloating, and pain levels can also provide useful clues.

Gradually reintroduce foods after a flare-up to pinpoint specific triggers. This process, called an elimination diet, involves removing certain foods for a period, then slowly adding them back one at a time, observing your body's response. This helps identify which foods may be irritating your digestive system.

In addition to monitoring your diet, consider portion sizes. Eating large meals or eating too quickly can overwhelm your digestive system, leading to discomfort. Smaller, more frequent meals may be easier on your stomach, particularly during a flare-up or recovery phase.

Managing stress and staying hydrated are equally important in managing symptoms. Dehydration can aggravate digestive issues, while stress can trigger flare-ups. Practice stress-reduction techniques like deep breathing, meditation, or yoga to help keep your symptoms in check.

Finally, consult with your healthcare provider. They can help guide you in identifying food triggers, adjusting your diet, and making necessary lifestyle changes to manage diverticulitis symptoms.

Living Well with Diverticulitis

Living well with diverticulitis involves a combination of proactive health management, lifestyle adjustments, and consistent monitoring of symptoms. By embracing healthy habits and being mindful of how your body responds to different foods and activities, you can maintain a good quality of life while managing this condition.

Start by focusing on a balanced, anti-inflammatory diet. This includes foods that promote gut health and reduce inflammation, such as fiber-rich fruits, vegetables, lean proteins, and healthy fats like olive oil and nuts. However, during flare-ups, it's crucial to adjust your diet to easier-to-digest, low-residue foods to give your digestive system time to heal. Be sure to avoid common triggers and gradually reintroduce foods to test your tolerance.

Regular physical activity is another key to managing diverticulitis. Low-impact exercises like walking, yoga, and swimming can promote healthy digestion and reduce stress, which can be a significant trigger for flare-ups. Staying hydrated is also essential, as it helps keep the digestive system functioning optimally and prevents constipation.

Stress management is vital for long-term health. Stress can exacerbate symptoms, so finding ways to relax and unwind, whether through meditation, breathing exercises, or mindfulness practices, can have a significant impact on how well you manage your condition. Ensuring you get adequate rest and sleep is equally important in maintaining your body's overall health.

Tracking your symptoms and progress regularly allows you to understand your triggers and make informed decisions about your lifestyle and diet. Always stay in communication with your healthcare provider to ensure you're on the right track and to make necessary adjustments to your treatment plan.

By adopting a holistic approach to managing diverticulitis and prioritizing your health, you can enhance your quality of life and reduce the frequency and severity of flare-ups.

Glossary of Digestive-Friendly Ingredients

1. Aloe Vera
A soothing plant known for its anti-inflammatory properties. Aloe vera juice or gel can be used to support digestion and reduce irritation in the gastrointestinal tract.

2. Bananas
Easily digestible, bananas are high in potassium and soluble fiber, making them ideal for soothing the stomach during digestive distress.

3. Bone Broth
A nutrient-dense liquid made by simmering animal bones. It is rich in collagen, gelatin, and amino acids that support gut health, reduce inflammation, and promote healing.

4. Coconut Oil
A healthy fat that is easy to digest and known for its antimicrobial properties. Coconut oil can help

soothe the digestive tract and provide a source of energy for the body.

5. Ginger
A natural anti-inflammatory and digestive aid. Ginger can help reduce nausea, bloating, and discomfort associated with digestive issues.

6. Oats
A soluble fiber source that promotes healthy digestion. Oats are gentle on the stomach and can help regulate bowel movements and reduce inflammation.

7. Papaya
A tropical fruit rich in the enzyme papain, which aids digestion by breaking down proteins. It also contains anti-inflammatory properties and supports gut health.

8. Rice
A low-fiber food that is easy on the stomach, particularly when made into a porridge or soup. Rice

is often recommended during flare-ups as part of a bland diet.

9. Sweet Potatoes
A rich source of vitamins, fiber, and antioxidants. Sweet potatoes are gentle on the stomach and can provide soothing relief during digestive distress.

10. Yogurt (with probiotics)
Yogurt that contains live cultures can help restore balance to the gut microbiota. Probiotics found in yogurt support digestion and may reduce the risk of flare-ups in individuals with diverticulitis.

11. Zucchini
A soft, low-fiber vegetable that is easy to digest. Zucchini is a great choice for cooking during recovery or flare-up phases, as it provides hydration and nutrients without irritating the digestive system.

12. Chamomile
A calming herb that can help reduce inflammation and soothe the digestive tract. Chamomile tea is

often used to relieve bloating, indigestion, and stomach cramps.

13. Spinach

When cooked, spinach is a soft, nutrient-rich vegetable that is high in vitamins A, C, and K, as well as folate. It can be easy to digest when cooked until tender.

14. Carrots

Carrots are a gentle vegetable on the digestive system when cooked and pureed. They are rich in beta-carotene and fiber, making them great for promoting gut health while being gentle during flare-ups.

15. Lentils

A source of plant-based protein and fiber that is easy to digest when well-cooked. Lentils can be a great addition to meals once you're in the recovery phase, supporting digestive health with gentle fiber.

16. Turmeric

An anti-inflammatory spice that contains curcumin, known for its digestive benefits. Turmeric can help reduce inflammation in the gut and promote overall digestive comfort.

17. Cucumber
A hydrating vegetable that is easy on the digestive system when peeled and served in soft preparations. Cucumbers are high in water and low in fiber, making them soothing for the stomach.

18. Fennel
A digestive aid that can reduce bloating and gas. Fennel seeds or tea are commonly used to relieve digestive discomfort and promote smooth digestion.

19. Paprika
A mild spice made from dried peppers. It can add flavor to meals without irritating the digestive tract, making it a good choice for individuals with diverticulitis when used in moderation.

20. Flaxseeds

A source of soluble fiber that helps with digestion and promotes regular bowel movements. Flaxseeds are often ground and added to smoothies or baked goods to support digestive health.

These ingredients are gentle on the digestive system and can be incorporated into a diet that supports healing, reduces inflammation, and promotes overall digestive health. Always consult with your healthcare provider to ensure that these ingredients are appropriate for your specific condition.

Kitchen Conversion Charts

Volume Conversions

1 teaspoon = 5 milliliters

1 tablespoon = 15 milliliters

1 fluid ounce = 30 milliliters

1 cup = 240 milliliters

1 pint = 480 milliliters

1 quart = 960 milliliters

1 gallon = 3.8 liters

Weight Conversions

1 ounce = 28 grams

1 pound = 454 grams

1 kilogram = 2.2 pounds

Temperature Conversions

Celsius to Fahrenheit: (°C × 9/5) + 32 = °F

Fahrenheit to Celsius: (°F - 32) × 5/9 = °C

Dry Ingredient Conversions

1 cup all-purpose flour = 120 grams

1 cup granulated sugar = 200 grams

1 cup brown sugar (packed) = 220 grams

1 cup powdered sugar = 120 grams

1 cup butter = 227 grams

1 large egg = approximately 50 grams

1 cup rolled oats = 90 grams

1 cup rice (uncooked) = 190 grams

1 cup lentils (uncooked) = 200 grams

Liquid Ingredient Conversions

1 cup = 240 milliliters

1 tablespoon = 15 milliliters

1 teaspoon = 5 milliliters

1 fluid ounce = 30 milliliters

1 pint = 473 milliliters

1 quart = 946 milliliters

1 gallon = 3.8 liters

Metric to US Measurements

1 liter = 4.2 cups

1 milliliter = 0.04 fluid ounces

1 kilogram = 2.2 pounds

1 gram = 0.035 ounces

Cooking and Baking Pan Size Conversions

9" round pan = 8 cups

8" square pan = 6 cups

9x13" pan = 14-16 cups

1 muffin cup = 1/4 cup

1 standard baking sheet = 15x10 inches

These conversion charts will help you navigate kitchen measurements, whether you're adjusting recipes, cooking, or baking with different ingredients. Keep them handy for accurate cooking and baking results!

Made in the USA
Middletown, DE
22 December 2024